Curriculum Development in Nursing

Process and Innovations

Leana R Uys and Nomthandazo S Gwele

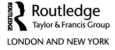

Routledge
Taylor & Francis Group

LONDON AND NEW YORK

First published in 2005 by Routledge
2 Park Square, Milton Park, Abingdon, Oxon OX14 4RN

Simultaneously published in the USA and Canada
by Routledge
29 West 35th Street, New York, NY 10001

Routledge is an imprint of the Taylor & Francis Group

Typeset in Sabon MT by J&L Composition, Filey, North Yorkshire
Printed and bound in Great Britain by TJ International Ltd,
Padstow, Cornwall

British Library Cataloguing in Publication Data
A catalogue record for this book is available from the British
Library

Library of Congress Cataloging in Publication Data
A catalogue record for this book has been requested

ISBN 0-415-34629-0 (hbk)
ISBN 0-415-34630-4 (pbk)

Contents

Preface

Nurse educators always have a dual role – they are both nurses and educators. As nurses they often have a specialty, such as psychiatric nursing or nephrology nursing, and they need to keep up with developments in that specialty, both in terms of the literature and the practice. When such nurses become educators, they also have to master the field of education, and keep up with what is new in the field of education, both in terms of theory and practice. We therefore believe that such nurse educators need constructive, stimulating and up-to-date texts to assist them in their task as educators of the new generation of nurses.

Nursing and midwifery are facing increasing demands the world over, but especially in developing countries. Healthcare quality is often dependent on the quality of nurses and midwives, since they provide the bulk of the human resource capacity. Their traditional hospital-based, lecturer-dependent and narrowly focused training often does little, however, to prepare them for the realities they face in practice in under-served areas, where they need to work and think independently, and where they need to lead the health team and the community. The fact that resources are often scarce, and support for nursing education compares poorly with that for medical education, does not help. The challenge is therefore often how to do more with less.

We, Leana and Thandi, have been active in our own country, and internationally, assisting nurse educators to interrogate their own curricula, their own teaching practice and their own views on nursing education. In many places we have found enthusiastic colleagues who want to deliver quality nursing education, but who are caught in old paradigms, and outdated methods. Often they have had limited exposure to higher education settings, but are expected to develop new nursing schools in universities. In such circumstances they often carry poor educational practices from other settings into new programmes and schools. Under pressure to develop new curricula fast with limited resources, and implement these curricula for groups of students used to traditional teaching/learning, they fall back on what they have been used to in their own school and nursing education.

As we worked in such settings over time, we often felt the need for a book that we could leave with them to assist them when we had left. We could find nothing that articulated our belief in innovative process-outcome curricula, based on solid preparation of the curriculum, staff and students. There was nothing that gave the simple information one needs when leading a nursing programme: how you plan for clinical learning experiences, how you decide how much clinical learning is enough, how you balance process with content and outcomes.

The purpose of this book is to offer nurse-educators a single textbook that brings together two aspects:

- the generic process, outlining each step carefully to support faculty who actually have to develop a curriculum, and
- innovative approaches which have developed over the last 20 years, and are still new to most nurse-educators.

This book gives enough detail to enable a group of nurse educators to use it to work through the process of developing a curriculum. It is a 'how to' guide, but it outlines adequately the theoretical and philosophical reasoning behind the decisions made. It also gives more detail of specific types of innovative curricula, to support groups who want to implement such models. Since most of the authors are second-language English speakers, the writing is usually easy to understand, and is also illustrated with examples, both in the text and in the form of recommended readings.

Chapter 1 provides a philosophical basis for the process of curriculum development, and anchors the more practical chapters which follow.

Chapters 2–7 deal with the process of curriculum development, implementation and evaluation. In each chapter one step of the process is described, explaining what it entails, and how the educators should go about completing the tasks.

Chapters 8–13 give examples of the more common types of innovative curricula. In each case the author deals with the characteristics of the specific type of curriculum, the advantages and disadvantages, and then describes the specific tasks involved in developing such a curriculum. The specifics about the implementation of each kind of curriculum are also given, and often the author refers to a real life curriculum as an example. Since more than one type of curriculum uses cases of problem-scenarios, one chapter (Chapter 10) is dedicated to the development of such components. Problem-based, case-based, outcomes-based, community-based and interprofessional learning are all innovations that have built up some credibility over the last 20 years, but can still all be seen as innovative.

At the end of each chapter we recommend a few readings which give examples of either research done in the topic covered by the chapter, or give a description of implementation of the topic of the chapter. For instance, at the end of Chapter 6 on the implementation of a new curriculum, one article describes an example of such an implementation process, while the other describes a research project on staff concerns during the implementation project. We also list one or two points for discussion, to assist groups to engage around the issues raised in the chapter. Having read and studied the chapter the reader might be stimulated by these points to apply the new knowledge, or search further for answers.

Curriculum development is something all the authors of this book feel passionately about. We hope that the book will stimulate readers to create something new in nursing and midwifery education, and to facilitate the creation of a new cadre of nurses and midwives who can confidently lead us towards the ideal of 'Health for All'.

Leana Uys and Nomthandazo Gwele
Durban, March, 2005

Contributors

Henry Y Akinsola is a registered nurse and a registered nurse tutor. He trained in Nigeria as a diploma nurse in 1973. He did his first degree (B.Sc. in Nursing, 1978) and PhD in Community Health (1991) at the University of Ibadan, Nigeria. He holds the degree Master of Science in Community Medicine from the University of Manchester, England (1983). He has been involved in the training of nurses and doctors for the past 21 years, having worked in Universities in several African countries, including Nigeria, Kenya and Botswana. Currently he is the team leader of project designed to integrate quality assurance principles in the nursing training curricula of the College of Nursing and Health Technology, Ministry of Health, Asmara, Eritrea.

Nomthandazo S Gwele (Thandi) is a registered nurse and midwife, and a registered nurse educator. She started her nursing career in a Diploma programme at Frere Hospital in East London, South Africa. While working as a midwife and a community health nurse, she obtained her BA (Nursing) in 1984 from the University of South Africa. In 1985 she travelled to the USA on a bursary, and obtained both the M Education and the MS (Nursing) at the University of Missouri-Columbia before returning to South Africa. Having worked at the University of Transkei, she joined the staff of the University of Natal (now KwaZulu-Natal) in 1992, where she obtained her PhD in 1994. Over the last 10 years she has acted as curriculum consultant to numerous nursing colleges and universities in South Africa, she also worked closely with the Nursing Institute of the United Arab Emirates. She was Head of the School of Nursing at the University of KwaZulu-Natal, Durban, South Africa.

Marilyn R Lee began her nursing career in 1971 as a Staff Nurse after completing her Diploma in Nursing at the Barnes Hospital School of Nursing in St. Louis, Missouri, USA. She was Head Nurse, Clinical Nurse and Inservice Instructor there over the next 10 years. She subsequently obtained BSN (1976) and BA (1975) from the University of St. Louis and her M Nursing (1982) from the University of South Carolina. In 1983 she taught in the School of Nursing at McMaster University, where for the next 16 years she taught nursing students using problem- and case-based approaches to learning in Canada and later in Pakistan. While in Pakistan, she was coordinator and team leader in two projects in nursing education and leadership development. She received her PhD in Nursing from Wayne State University, Detroit, Michigan, USA in 1996. In 1999 she moved to the University of Botswana (in Gabarone), where she is currently the first Deputy Director in the new Academic Programme Review Unit.

Fikile Mtshali is a registered nurse and midwife, and also registered operating room nurse, nurse educator and nurse administrator. She has worked in a range of clinical settings for many years before embarking on an academic career. She obtained her PhD in 2003 with a study on Community-based Education in nursing in South Africa. She has been working as a consultant in different African countries, including Rwanda and Tanzania, as part of the work of the School of Nursing at the University of KwaZulu-Natal. She is currently Post-graduate Programme Director in the School of Nursing, University of KwaZulu-Natal, Durban, South Africa.

Mouzza Suwaileh graduated from the B.Sc Nursing programme in the College of Health Sciences in 1987, and also has a qualification in health professional education from the same institution. She obtained an M.Sc in Adult Health Nursing from the University of Texas Medical Branch in Galveston in 1990 and then a PhD in Nursing from the University of Texas in Austin, USA. She also did a Diploma in Health Care Management from Royal College of Surgeons, Ireland in 2002. She worked in various units in Bahrain hospitals, and is a certified haemodialysis nurse. She is currently the Chairperson of the Nursing Division at the College of Health Sciences, Kingdom of Bahrain, and the Director of WHO Collaborating Center for Nursing Development, Kingdom of Bahrain.

Leana R Uys is a registered nurse and midwife, and also a registered psychiatric nurse, nurse educator and nurse administrator. She started her nursing career by doing a B Nursing at the University of Pretoria in South Africa, and joined the University of the Free State after spending 2 years in a rural hospital. There she did her Masters (1975) and D.Soc.Sc (1980), and also an Honours degree in Psychology (1973) and another in Philosophy (1984). In 1986 she joined the School of Nursing at the University of Natal (now KwaZulu-Natal) as Head, and led the change of the nursing programme from a traditional curriculum to a problem-based learning and community-based education curriculum during the 1990s. When the school became a WHO Collaborating Centre for Nursing and Midwifery development in Africa in 1996, she became the first Director of this centre. She has written a number of nursing textbooks, and has been an active researcher in nursing education. She is currently Executive Dean of Health Sciences of the University of KwaZulu-Natal, Durban, South Africa.

Abbreviations

AACN	American Association of Colleges of Nursing
CBAM	Concerns-based Adoption Model
CBE	Community-based education
CBL	Case-based learning
CIPP	Context-Input-Process-Product
IPL	Inter-professional learning
MPL	Multi-professional learning
OBE	Outcomes-based education
PBL	Problem-based learning
PHC	Primary health care
SDL	Self-directed learning
UNFPA	United Nations Population Fund
WHO	World Health Organization
ZPD	Zone of Proximal Development

Glossary

Case A comprehensive description of a clinical or practical case, which may be an individual, a group, a setting, or an organization, used as the basis for teaching or learning. In this text, it is used mainly with regard to the case-based curriculum.

Case-based curriculum (CBC) A curriculum in which students are given a set of complete cases for study and research in preparation for subsequent class discussions.

Course A building block of a programme, consisting of a time-limited component, usually over one term (3 months), one semester (6 months) or 1 year, and usually ending with a summative evaluation.

Community The community is regarded as a learning space in which students are exposed to live dynamic contexts, conscientizing them to the socio-economic, political, cultural and other factors influencing the health of individuals, families and the public at large.

Community-based education (CBE) A curriculum which focuses on learning activities that utilize the community extensively as a learning environment in which not only the students, but also the teachers, members of the community, and representatives of other sectors are actively involved throughout the educational experience.

Competence The ability to deliver a specified professional service.

Course outline A brief description of a course which allows the reader to understand the curriculum.

Curriculum Planned learning experiences offered in a single programme.

Curriculum strand   A repetitive idea or concept which appears throughout the curriculum and forms the framework for the choice of content and learning experiences.

Discipline   A field of study and practice often associated with a specific profession, or the group of scientists studying a specific subject.

Head of School   The Head of School is the person, usually a nurse, who is the executive director of the school. The title might be Dean, Principal, Professor, but the job is to give academic and administrative leadership.

Interprofessional learning (IPL)   Educational approaches in which disciplines collaborate in the learning process to foster interprofessional interactions that enhance the practice of all disciplines involved.

Learning opportunity   A learning situation created by a nurse educator for a student to use to achieve a learning outcome.

Level (of a programme)   A period during which the subjects or courses taken are at a similar level of difficulty, at the end of which a decision is usually made about the progression of the student, based on comprehensive assessment of performance.

Macro-curriculum   The overall design or blueprint of the programme, done by a Curriculum Committee.

Micro-curriculum   The course outlines and unit plans, usually developed by the individual teacher.

Mission statement   A mission statement is a relatively permanent and broad statement of the objectives of an organization, distinguishing it from other similar organizations, and illustrating the main reason(s) for its existence.

Module   A unit within a programme or a course, which can be examined separately (modular instruction) or at the end of the course.

Occupational map   A document that identifies the role components of the group of nurses being prepared by the programme. For each role component, the map describes the competencies that make up the role.

Outcome   A relatively self-contained achievement, describing the expectations of a particular work role which acts as a benchmark against which individual performance is judged.

Outcomes-based education (OBE)   A competency-oriented, performance-based approach to education which is aimed at aligning education with the demands of the workplace, and at the same time develops transferable life skills, such as problem-solving and critical thinking skills.

Post-registration programmes   Offered to people who are already nurses or midwives, to equip them for a specialized field of practice.

Pre-registration programmes   Those programmes which non-nurses take to become nurses.

Problem-based learning (PBL)   An approach to learning and instruction in which students tackle problems in small groups, under the supervision of a teacher or facilitator.

Programme   A coherent set of courses, leading to a certain degree, diploma or certificate. Courses might be core (compulsory) or optional courses (electives).

Regulatory body   Usually a statutory body established to maintain the standards of a profession by a range of activities, which usually include keeping a list (register) of practitioners who meet the required standard of education and practice.

Scenario   A brief description of a clinical or practical case that is relevant to the learner, used as the basis for teaching or learning. In this text it is used mainly with regard to problem-based learning, and is used interchangeably with 'vignette'.

School of Nursing   A department within a university, or a college or any other higher education institution that is in charge of offering formal nursing and midwifery programmes. It may also refer to the total higher education institution, in the case of a single-discipline institution.

Situation analysis   A comprehensive study of the context which shapes a school of nursing and its programmes.

Stakeholders   Individuals or groups who have an interest in the outcomes of an endeavour.

Subject   A clearly identifiable area of knowledge that studies a specific set of phenomena from a particular perspective, often using unique research methods.

Unit   The building block of a course, used interchangeably with 'module'.

Chapter 1

Education philosophy and the curriculum

Nomthandazo S Gwele

Introduction

The term curriculum means many things to many people. Any attempt to define the concept within the context of this chapter is not aimed at seeking consensus of interpretation but rather an understanding of the meaning attached to the concept in the context of this book. Curriculum here refers to planned learning experiences that the educational institution intends to provide for its learners. This definition does not deny the existence of hidden and null curricula (that which the educational institution chooses to exclude from its curriculum (Eisner, 1994), in educational institutions, but is seen as an appropriate point of departure for a book on curriculum development, since what is not planned or cannot be planned would be difficult to articulate in such a book.

Despite the lack of agreement on the meaning of the term, there seems to be consensus that educational institutions, as institutions charged with the all important societal function of educating citizens, have the sole claim to curriculum. Furthermore, most agree that in education of all forms, there is no such thing as being neutral (Bode, 1937; Moore, 2000; Smeyers, 1995). Some authors believe that education should be directed towards helping learners become intelligent and critical citizens in a democratic society (Dewey, 1916, 1961); yet for some, education is a political act that 'demands from educators that they take it on as a political act and that they consistently live their progressive and democratic or authoritarian and reactionary past or also their spontaneous, uncritical choice, that they define themselves by being democratic or authoritarian' (Freire, 1998: 63). Put simply, either the learners have to be taught to fit as a cog into the existing social machinery, or to recognize their own responsibility for the transformation of the social, political and economic world in which they live (Bode, 1937). In Cuffaro's words 'philosophy of education represents choices, values, knowledge and beliefs of teachers as well as their aspirations, intentions and aims. It serves to guide and inspire and contributes to determining the detail of every day life in the classroom' (1994: 1).

Central to making educational choices is a need to make explicit the philosophical beliefs underpinning what the educational institution sees as worthwhile for learners to experience. Such beliefs, whether made explicit or not, permeate the curricula experiences of all the learners in whatever context they find themselves. As noted by Wiles and Bondi 'at the heart of purposeful activity in curriculum development is an educational philosophy that assists in answering value-laden questions and selecting from among the many choices' (1998: 35). This is specifically true about choices and questions related to the purpose of education, the nature and role of the learner, the nature and role of the teacher and the teaching/learning process.

Choices and decisions about curriculum are, hopefully, not random choices, but are based on thorough understanding of the educational ideologies on which they are based. Three broad streams of educational philosophy underpin curricula choices and decisions; the conservative, the progressive and the radical views. It should be noted, however, that most of what has been written in educational philosophy has been directed to formative education, that is, that aspect of education that takes place during the years of primary and secondary education. For some reason, it seems that educational philosophers have preferred to stay clear of tertiary education, especially professional education. On the other hand, educators in the professions have been drawn to the philosophical debates underlying their practice.

The conservative view

The basic premise underpinning the conservative vision is that there are certain enduring worthwhile truths that should be taught and learned. According to this view, the purpose of education is to transmit worthwhile bodies of information to generations of learners so that that which is worthwhile is conserved. Two schools of thought, perennialism and essentialism, fall within the conservative vision. Although the two schools of thought differ somewhat in how they view education, they agree on various fundamental aspects about education. For both the perennialists and the essentialists, education should concern itself with the cultivation of the intellect and not learner needs or interests (Tanner and Tanner, 1995). Furthermore, the two schools of thought agree that:

- social change should be slow
- there is need to conserve and therefore to oppose reform
- methodology should be teacher directed
- emphasis should be placed on ensuring content-centred curriculum (Hearne and Cowles, 2001: 54).

Differences between the two schools of thought revolve around specifications of exactly what is to be taught and for what purpose. Perennialists' views of education have limited relevance to professional education because of their focus on the basics such as the reading, writing and arithmetic. Hence, this chapter focuses mainly on a brief analysis of the essentialists' view of education.

The decision to focus mainly on essentialism is not to negate the tight grip that perennialists' views on education have had on nursing education in particular. It has been noted that 'perennialists contend that there is an organized body of knowledge that children (learners – insertion mine) need to know so that society might cohere around a common identity' (Gaudelli, 2002: 198). That nursing education has always largely been, and continues to be, in many parts of the world a content-driven and transmission-dominated educational system is by no means an accident. The biomedical approach, and its foundational sciences in the form of applied medical sciences, continue to dominate what is learned in nursing schools globally. Attempts to marginalize the concepts of disease and the pathophysiological processes affecting body organs and systems, through the introduction of integrated curricula in nursing education have not been very successful. Regulatory nursing organizations implicitly or explicitly continue to demand clear indications of how much medical nursing, surgical nursing, paediatric nursing or obstetric and gynaecological nursing a prospective practising nurse has been exposed to during her/his period of education and training. The pervasive and enduring quality of perennialism in education, including professional education, cannot be underestimated. Admittedly, this is not the list of topics that one would find in the Great Books of western civilization, but it is a list of topics that one would find in western medical and/or nursing textbooks.

Essentialism

Rooted in idealism and realism, essentialists contend that both body and mind are important in education and as such 'core knowledge and skills are essential to a successful society, because those requisite abilities allow the individual to be an economically productive member of society' (Gaudelli, 2002: 198). Four broad presuppositions that underpin essentialism are identified by Gaudelli (2002: 199) as follows:

- human nature tends to be bad
- culture is outside the individual
- consciousness should be focused on the present and the future
- the centre of value is found in the body and to a lesser degree in the mind.

The mind, however, has value in so far as it can be manipulated, cultivated and moulded to deal with the demands of an academically demanding education. In the words of Tanner and Tanner 'like the perennialist, the essentialist conceives of the mind as a vessel or container. Individual differences are marked off according to mental capacities, and education is simply a matter of filling and stretching each mind with the same curricular brew to the utmost of each mind's capacity' (1995: 314).

The purpose of education

The purpose of education, from the essentialists' perspective, is the preservation, through transmission to generations of learners, of that which is essential to learn. The goal of education is to instil in learners the academic and moral knowledge which should constitute those 'essential things that a mature adult needs to know in order to be a productive member of society' (Hearne and Cowles, 2001: 54). There is no doubt that education is the most contested sector in any country. Power and politics often dictate which path in education will hold sway at any point in time in any part of the world. Ernest (1991) refers to present-day essentialism as technological pragmatism, in which absolutist epistemological views about education are based on the values of utilitarianism, expediency, wealth creation and technological development.

The curriculum

For the essentialists, knowledge is not to be found only in the Great Books of the western world, but is likely to be found in a variety of places. For them, knowledge is what is real and reality exists outside the individual and is subject to observation. Nevertheless, similar to the perennialists, the essentialists are of the view that only certain subjects are capable of cultivating the intellect; and therefore essential for the school to realize its purpose. These are 'the fundamental academic disciplines of English (grammar, literature and composition), mathematics, science, history and modern languages. . . . The performing arts, industrial arts, vocational studies, physical education and other areas of the curriculum are regarded as frills' (Tanner and Tanner, 1995: 313). The essentialists do admit, however, that core knowledge and skills might change over time, depending on what is essential to know in order to function as a mature and productive adult both in the present and in the future. According to this view, a curriculum cannot be based on learners' needs and wants, but rather on what those in authority know is essential for the learners to know.

Nature and role of the learner

From the essentialist perspective, the learner is seen as a passive recipient of information transmitted by disciplinary experts. The learner's role is not to reason why, but to do as told. The interests and needs of the learner are seen as irrelevant to the educative process. What is important, though, is the conviction that learners differ greatly in their mental capabilities, and that it is not the function of the education system or the school to provide what the learner's genes have failed to provide. Hence the emphasis on ability grouping and testing to weed out those who can from those who just can't.

Nature and role of the teacher

The teacher knows best. The teacher is an expert with a wealth of information which he/she must transmit to the learner. It is therefore his/her duty to ensure that all that is essential to learn is taught. The teacher is charged with the responsibility to identify, select and organize that which is to be learned, and to decide how and when it is to be learned.

The nature of the teaching/learning process

For the essentialists, learning is no more than acquisition of knowledge and skills. According to this perspective this acquisition is best achieved through a teaching/learning process that places emphasis on lectures, drill, recitation and demonstration, provided and led by an expert in the discipline. Mastery has to be demonstrated through performance in various forms of assessment. In fact essentialists are credited for the proliferation of standardized tests and assessment in the USA (Tanner and Tanner, 1995)

The progressive view

Progressivism is associated with the rise in dissatisfaction with traditional education practices which placed emphasis on content and totally disregarded the place of learners' needs and interest in education. Two streams of progressive education are evident in the educational philosophy literature. The European stream, often referred to as 'child-centred' education based on Rousseau's fictitious teacher, and his equally fictitious pupil Emile, rebelled mainly against what was seen as over-subjugation of the pupil to conservative ideals propagated through traditional education. This stream is also sometimes called progressive romantic naturalism (Tanner and Tanner, 1995). The basic premise underpinning romantic naturalism (European progressivism) was that society interferes too much in the education of children. Children, if left alone, have the potential to grow up and become distinct and individual beings, untainted by societal influences and thinking. Each learner, therefore, is seen as a potential flower. In fact, Rousseau believed that the best that the teacher can do is do nothing (Tanner and Tanner, 1995). Closely related to romantic naturalism is existentialism. Advocates of existentialism proceed from the view that the world is an impersonal and indifferent place, and therefore, individuals must find their own meaning for existence because in their view 'existence precedes essence' (cited in Noddings, 1995: 59). Meaning for one's existence therefore, can only be found through freedom of choice and introspection. Existentialism and/or romantic education, has not had any significant influence in nursing education. For this reason, these two schools of thought will not be dealt with any further than the cursory reference they deserve in a chapter whose main focus is to provide a frame of reference for developing a nursing curriculum.

Progressive education in the United States had some tenets in common with its European counterpart, but was also very distinct in its view about the place of education and therefore the school in the society. John Dewey, a prominent and prolific writer in educational philosophy, is often referred to as the father of progressive education in the USA. Dewey's philosophy of education is often called pragmatism or experimentalism. From this perspective, education should not be isolated from its social context, because education and experience are inextricably intertwined. Education therefore, must focus on the learner's experiences and interests rather than on predetermined bodies of knowledge. This does not mean that content has no place in education, but rather that the learner's experience must be used to mediate knowledge.

Distinctions aside, a number of commonalities exist among the broad streams of progressive thought in education. From the progressives' perspective knowledge is not static but dynamic, and learner's interests and needs are just as important as the content to be learned. Experience is the best source of knowledge, rather than the textbook. Learners learn best by doing, experimenting and finding meaning in their own actions and in the consequences of decisions taken.

Experimentalism

The basic premise on which experimentalism is based is that reality is external and observable. Truth is only that which can be verified through experimental testing. The underlying philosophy on which this ideology is based is pragmatism. Pragmatists, such as Pierce, Dewey and Whitehead are of the view that what is real and true, is what works. Knowledge therefore, is judged on the basis of its consequences.

Broad presuppositions underpinning experimentalism include the following:

- the meaning and value of ideas is only found in practical results
- ideas must always be tested by experimentation
- change is the only constant in human existence
- the ability to adjust to and/or deal with change is fundamental to constructive and democratic living (Tanner and Tanner, 1995).

The purpose of education

It is worth noting at this point, that from Dewey's perspective, the man closely associated with progressive education, pragmatism and experimentalism in the USA, 'education as such has no aims' (1961: 107). Instead people, parents, teachers and governments have aims. From the experimentalist perspective, the purpose of education is to help learners make connections between their life experiences and the world of schooling. The level of experience and the learner's interest should therefore be the starting point in any educational event.

Education should help learners to become responsible and critical citizens in democratic societies. From the experimentalist perspective, and Dewey's in particular, education should be conceived as 'the development of the learner's capacities and interests in ways that empower her or him to assume the role of constructive participant in the life of the wider society' (Hickman, 1998: xv).

The curriculum

From the experimentalist's perspective, life experience should form the basis of what is learned, because experience consists of 'the active interrelationship between the external world and the individual, between the thing and its sensation, perception, image and idea; between the objective and subjective aspects of human life' (Novack, 1975: 161). Furthermore, because life has a scientific, aesthetic, and social aspect, the disciplines themselves are important only in so far as they are used to interpret the learner's experiences, rather than as lessons and/or information that has to be passively assimilated and stored for later use (Dewey, 1897, 1998: 233).

Nature and role of the learner

The learner is viewed as a psychological and social being. The psychological and social aspects of the learner are organically intertwined, and one does not take precedence over another (Dewey, 1998). Through the process of development, the learner is seen as constantly seeking to find meaning in the world around him/her. He/she is directed by interest evoked by images in his/her life world. This natural tendency to 'inquire', or to be curious, allows the learner to direct his or her actions to the pursuit of those experiences, and the answers arrived at lead to a better understanding of his/her world.

Nature and role of the teacher

From the experimentalist's perspective, the teacher, by virtue of his or her experience and wisdom, has a responsibility to 'assist the learner in properly responding to these experiences' (Dewey, 1998: 231). In essence, the teacher is viewed, not merely as a transmitter of knowledge and ideas, but mainly as a mediator of knowledge. It is the teacher who has to help the learner negotiate meaning from his/her experiences in the light of what is already known (subject matter or disciplines). In recent years, this view has led to extensive discourse on mediation of knowledge.

The nature of the teaching/learning process

Similar to all progressives, the experimentalists prefer learning by doing (experimentation) rather than passively listening to lectures. The basic premise is that ideas result from action (Dewey, 1998). Experiential learning and constructivism are the learning theories driving the teaching/learning process in experimentalist progressive classrooms. Grounded in the belief that knowledge is socially constructed in interaction with others, active learning approaches to teaching/learning are preferred. Hence, experimentalist classrooms are characterized by 'participation in meaningful projects, learning by doing, encountering problems and solving them, not only to facilitate acquisition and retention of knowledge but to foster the right character traits: usefulness, helpfulness, critical intelligence, individual initiative' (Novack, 1975: 228).

The radical view

Dissatisfied with the progressive educationists' pre-occupation with learners' needs and focus on education for participatory democracy, the advocates of radical education manifested themselves, initially, in the form of such celebrated educational philosophers and/or scholars as Harold Rugg, George Counts, Henry Giroux, Antonio Gramsci and Paulo Freire. Although not necessarily agreeing on every fundamental question about education, these philosophers were all of the view that education should do more than prepare learners for participatory democratic citizenship. Education should also prepare them for deliberative citizenship. The two prominent radical schools of thought in educational theory and/or philosophy that will be dealt with in this chapter are reconstructionism and critical curriculum theory (critical pedagogy).

Reconstructionism

Reconstructionism is commonly seen as a branch of progressive education. It is discussed under the radical vision in this chapter, because of its conception of education as a vehicle for effecting fundamental social change, especially in the realm of socio-political, economic and cultural organization. Central to reconstructionism is the conviction that societal change can be achieved through education (Kilgour, 1995). For reconstructionists, progressive education is too slow or too 'soft' ever to lead to change in the existing social order. Social and economic inequities cannot be solved through problem solving activities alone, but require constructive deliberations and even revolutionary action.

Two distinct groups within the reconstructionist school of thought exist: the ideological and the methodological. Ideological reconstructionism places emphasis on theory development and advances reconstructionism as a philosophy of action in education. Methodological reconstructionists, such as Ralph Tyler, place emphasis on advancing the application of research-based strategies for effecting social change in education (Weltman, 2002). Tyler (1949) identified four fundamental questions which must be answered in developing a curriculum and a plan of instruction, as follows:

- What educational purposes should the school seek to attain?
- What educational experiences can be provided that are likely to attain these purposes?
- How can these educational experiences be effectively organized?
- How can we determine whether these purposes are being attained?

In his view, information obtained from analysis of learner' needs, interests and characteristics, current life outside the school and views of subject experts should form the basis for making decisions about worthwhile educational purposes (Tyler, 1949). The basic principles of curriculum development, seen by others as the ultimate framework for a technocratic curriculum, were in fact intended as a broad and flexible tool for making sense of what is a complex and often overwhelming task for teachers, that is, the process of developing a curriculum (Tanner and Tanner, 1995). Despite widespread criticism of Tyler's principles for designing a curriculum, there is no denying the impact his work has had on nursing education. Tyler provided a framework for practitioners of education to help them find direction in the practice of curriculum development. Rhetoric and ideology help in getting teachers to begin to question their practice; principles and guidelines help teachers transform rhetoric into theory of practice, without which, even the most brilliant ideas are likely to founder.

The purpose of education

From the reconstructionists' perspective, the purpose of education is to 'reconstruct society through students' acquisition of problem-solving skills applied to real life' (Stern and Riley, 2002: 114). The basic premise here is that education, and therefore by implication the schools, should be used as instruments of social change. In the words of Rugg, 'we need of course to prepare our youth adequately to participate in life activities. . . . But we also need to prepare them to improve the situation in which they will find themselves as adults. We must equip them to be constructively critical of contemporary social, economic and political organization' (cited in Stern and Riley, 2002: 114).

As early as 1932, Counts had written that '[Education] . . . must . . . face squarely and courageously every social issue, come to grips with life in all of its stark reality, establish an organic relation with the community, develop a realistic and comprehensive theory of welfare, fashion a compelling and challenging vision of human destiny, and become less frightened than it is today at the bogies of imposition and indoctrination' (cited in Slattery, 1995: 195).

The curriculum

The social studies curriculum is preferred over other disciplines, such as natural sciences. Any discipline, however, is relevant in so far as it is used to interrogate the societal issues facing the learners and the society as a whole. The enduring societal issues, which no democracy or totalitarian society has ever succeeded in eliminating, such as equity of opportunity, access to education, political power and freedom from oppression are seen as central in a reconstructionist curriculum. A conscientizing and liberating curriculum is seen as most worthy of ensuring that education fulfils its purpose of changing the social order.

The nature and role of the teacher

From the reconstructionist perspective, teachers have to be courageous and bold in performing their roles in reconstructing. For Counts, even indoctrination and imposition of the liberation ideology by teachers was a necessary strategy which teachers should not be afraid to use. According to him, it is a fallacy that the school should be impartial, since 'schooling is complicit in forms of social control and indoctrination that result in social injustices' (cited in Slattery, 1995: 195).

The nature and role of the learner

Tanner and Tanner describe an ideal learner within the social reconstructionist perspective as a 'rebel committed to and involved in constructive social redirection and renewal' (1995: 305). The role of the learner therefore, is to understand and rebel against those forces that operate to create and maintain social, economic and political inequities. Assimilation of revolutionary rhetoric is what learners are expected to do. For reconstructionists such as Counts and Brameld, this was to be achieved by whatever means, whether by indoctrination or reason (Tanner and Tanner, 1995).

The nature of the teaching/learning process

Social reconstructionist classrooms as conceived by Counts and other reconstructionist scholars of the time, would not have differed much from the essentialist classrooms. What was taught would have been different rather than what was expected of the learners. Indoctrination and imposition would not have left any room for questioning on the part of the learners. The expectation would be that the learners would accept that what was taught was true and that they themselves had a responsibility to reconstruct the society, through revolutionary actions and/or legislation. Cooperative and collaborative learning experiences with the community as a starting point are seen as the best approaches to helping learners develop a sense of self and community awareness (Reed and Davis, 1999). Creating connections between the classroom and the community has a potential to evoke a strong emotional response from the learner, an ideal condition for indoctrination.

Critical curriculum theory

Revived in the works of contemporary educational philosophers such as Henry Giroux, and spurred by the failure of early 20th century revolutionary education as advocated by Counts and his associates, interest in education as an instrument of social change has again begun to dominate educational and/or curriculum discourse. The point of departure for critical curriculum theorists is that 'schools (and by implication education – insertion mine) contribute to cultural reproduction of class relations and economic order that allows very little social mobility' (Slattery, 1995: 193). Within the variants of critical theory and its advocates, general assumptions on which this school of thought is based are apparent:

- all thought and power relations are inexorably linked
- these power relations form oppressive social arrangements
- facts and values are inseparable and are inscribed by ideology
- language is a key element in the formation of subjective identities, and thus critical literacy – the ability to negotiate passages through social systems and structures – is more important than functional literacy – the ability to decode and compute
- oppression is based in the reproduction of privileged knowledge codes and practices (Kincheloe and Pinar, cited in Slattery, 1995: 193).

The purpose of education

The advocates of critical curriculum theory conceive the purpose of education as enabling 'students to become transformers of society . . . (enabling) students to be critical thinkers and critics of society who are able to make decisions and take actions which will better the society in which they live' (21st Century Schools, 2004: 1). Giroux raises an important question in asking: 'whether schools should uncritically serve and reproduce the existing society or challenge the social order to develop and advance its democratic imperatives' (1988: 197). According to him, the goals of critical theory in education are to assess the emerging forms of capitalism and domination, and rethink and transform the meaning of human emancipation through a process of self-conscious critique. That education is a political act was explicit in Paulo Freire's (1972) work, through his now famous book, *Pedagogy of the Oppressed*. Freire reiterated the earlier reconstructionists' concerns with the domesticating and oppressive nature of what he called the 'banking concept' of education. This type of education forces learners to sit passively, listen and regurgitate what the teacher tells them without questioning.

The curriculum

Critical curriculum content is chosen, not on the basis of what is intrinsically worthwhile knowledge, but rather on the basis of social worth (Dewey, 1916, 1961). According to him a curriculum which acknowledges the social responsibilities of education must present situations where problems are relevant to the problems of living together, and where observations and information are calculated to develop social insight and interest. For the proponents of critical curriculum theory, when selecting knowledge for inclusion in the curriculum, a number of fundamental questions need to be asked:

- What knowledge is important for students to learn, in whose point of view and based on what?
- What knowledge is excluded and why?

Any curriculum selected without answering these questions is seen as suspect. Mason (2000) argues that it is widely accepted that 'the truth status' of any knowledge determines its inclusion in or exclusion from a curriculum. What is in dispute, however, is who should be making decisions about the selection of material for inclusion in or exclusion from the curriculum. Some critical curriculum theorists differentiate between 'technical knowledge, which can be measured and quantified; practical knowledge, which is geared toward helping individuals understand social events that are ongoing and situational; and emancipatory knowledge, which attempts to reconcile and transcend the opposition between technical and practical knowledge' (Habermas, in Slattery, 1995: 202). Above all, from the critical curriculum theorists' point of view, because knowledge is only created within a dialogical community and preferably, one in which differences of opinion are not only allowed but encouraged, curriculum content must be selected on the basis of meaningfulness and relevance for the society (Beyer, 1986).

The nature and role of the teacher

Critical curriculum theorists believe that it is the role and responsibility of the teacher to help learners learn how to think, and provide them with the tools they need in order to transform the society. From this perspective, teachers are seen as critical mediators of knowledge (Mason, 2000). The teacher's role then requires that he/she make accessible to the learners the culture, worldview, social arrangements, and everyday practices of their society in all of their subtleties and nuances so that the learners can begin to question that which they had always taken for granted (Mason, 2000). Teachers are expected to create spaces for learners to negotiate and interpret meaning from, and implications of, information for a diverse society.

The nature and role of the learner

The learner is conceived of as a critical and questioning individual. According to Slattery (1995), self-conscious critique is an essential element of critical theory. The role of the learner therefore is constantly to question the world in which he/she lives with a view to transformative action.

The teaching/learning process

Problem-posing and problem-solving educational experiences form the hallmark of a liberating education (Freire, 1972). Through posing questions based on contemporary problems of inequity, oppression, dominant cultures, and politics of race and class, teachers help learners reflect on these issues so that they can begin to understand the situation in which they live, so as to be able to effect change. In such classrooms textbooks only serve as tools for interpretation and analysis, rather than as authoritative sources of information. Debates, questioning (often Socratic in nature), and conversation are the teaching methodologies of choice.

Implications for designing a nursing curriculum

It seems apparent that this chapter has reached a point where the reader might ask, so what? An exploration of educational ideologies within the context of a book on curriculum development in nursing education is essential, for the simple reason that 'our professional philosophy must cohere with our overall philosophy of education, in particular post-compulsory and tertiary education . . .' (Walker, 1995: 81). Educational change in nursing will always be nationally and politically driven. National governments and national regulatory bodies will always have a dominant say in the direction which nursing education should take. Curriculum change, on the other hand, is the responsibility of the individual nursing education institution.

Three distinct and conflicting approaches to curriculum, content-driven, process-based and outcomes-based, continue to dominate literature on curriculum development. Table 1.1 depicts these three broad approaches to curriculum development and the value positions underpinning them. Each approach, as the name implies, proceeds from the point of view that content, process or outcome is the most worthwhile component in the curriculum. A content-driven curriculum is rooted on the essentialist traditions of the conservative view of education. As noted earlier, from an essentialist perspective, an accumulated body of knowledge exists for most disciplines, which is essential for learners to know.

The content-focused approach is the most widely used approach to designing a curriculum in nursing. The starting point for such a curriculum is usually a list of content areas that must be taught, often starting from the foundational

Table 1.1 Curriculum approaches and underlying value positions within the context of a nursing education program

	Content-based approach	Process-based approach	Outcomes-based approach
Underpinning educational philosophy	Essentialism and perennialism	Experimentalism	Reconstructionism (methodological)* Critical curriculum theory
Purpose of nursing education	Transmission of worthwhile bodies of accumulated nursing knowledge	Understanding of the world of nursing as inextricably intertwined with the world in which we live. Democratic participation in health policy issues	Reconstruction of the social order through critical understanding of social, political and economic determinants of health and disease Fostering commitment to collective reflection and action for change in the health status of the community Attainment of transformative work-related outcomes (competencies) for both individual and societal survival
Curriculum	Fundamental academic disciplines (anatomy, physiology, social sciences). Core nursing subjects (medical and surgical nursing, mental health nursing, etc.)	Learners' experiences of the world of nursing, health and disease presented in the form of health problems and/or case studies	Social, economic, and political issues affecting the health of the people Focus on social reconstruction as a health promotion strategy
Nature and role of the teacher	Expert in the discipline who must identify, select, organize and transmit worthwhile knowledge and/or information to the learner	A mediator of knowledge, through questioning and making accessible those experiences which are deemed to have a potential to facilitate the students' understanding of their professional role and functions as nurses	A consciousness raiser and a critical mediator of knowledge through creating spaces for critical reflection and action

	Content-based approach	Process-based approach	Outcomes-based approach
Nature and role of the learner	A passive and willing recipient of information	Psychological and social beings with a natural need to make connections between their experiences as students of nursing and the world in	Social and psychological beings at one with their community Their role is questioning and challenging the status, e.g. questioning and reflection on issues which they live such as why HIV/AIDS is a death knell for the poor, while the rich seem rarely to die from this disease; who has money for drugs and who does not and why, are all seen as legitimate issues which a nursing student should confront
The teaching/ learning process	Teacher-directed with emphasis on knowledge acquisition methodologies such as drill, lecture and demonstration. The driving learning theory is information-processing theory	Experience-based learning with emphasis on methodologies that promote active learning, problem solving, cooperative and collaborative learning and experimentation	Issue-based learning with emphasis on a preference for socio-cultural approaches to mediated action. Debates, Socratic questioning, simulations and conversations are the methodologies of choice

*It is believed that it is the nature of the stated outcomes rather than the approach itself that determines whether a curriculum would be seen as techno-behaviourist or behavioural- and growth-focused (see Weltman, 2002, and Tanner and Tanner, 1995: 267).

biomedical sciences and social sciences, followed by body systems. Most nursing programs the world over are still content-based in nature, probably because most nurse educators were educated in this manner. This type of curriculum is often described as the traditional curriculum model (Wellard and Edwards, 1999). Even when the subjects are integrated and taught by multidisciplinary teams, the basic approach to the curriculum is still usually content-based. Lectures, interspersed with discussions, dominate the teaching/learning process.

Learners are expected to assimilate what is taught and be able to recall it when required to do so in examinations.

The process-based curricula, on the other hand, focuses on helping learners learn how to learn. The basic premise is that there is too much knowledge available and that educational institutions, including nursing education institutions, have but a limited time to prepare students for a lifetime of professional work. The best that the teachers can do is help students learn how to locate information, analyse and interpret it, in order to solve life problems. Rooted in Dewey's progressive education ideology, especially his experimentalist and/or pragmatist approach, process-focused curricula emphasize development of life skills such as problem solving, critical thinking and democratic citizenship. In nursing education, problem-based learning has become a dominant approach in the process-focused curriculum. Experiential learning is the learning theory that informs this curriculum approach. The starting point is life experience, and authentic nursing situations, rather than topics for study or discussion. It is hoped that in the process of trying to understand and/or solve the problem through hypothesis generation and seeking alternative solutions, students will acquire skills to deal with both current and future life and professional situations.

Outcomes-based education (OBE) is very difficult to pin down in terms of its philosophical foundations. There are those who believe that it is based on the essentialist perspective because OBE like the content-driven curriculum proceeds from the premise that in worthwhile education some things are essential to be learned. Nevertheless, OBE within an essentialist perspective proceeds from defining the standards or outcomes which must be attained by every learner seeking a particular qualification. Alexander refers to the latter view of OBE as a technological pragmatic view of education rather than essentialist (cited in Gross et al., 2003).

From the perspective of this chapter, guided by the author's interpretations, OBE is seen as a radical view of education, albeit a centrally designed mandated one. The main aim of OBE is social reconstruction. Properly implemented, OBE has the potential to lead to critical learners, learners who view education as more than acquisition of knowledge and skills for solving life problems, who 'understand how social relationships are distorted and manipulated by relations of power and privilege' (Slattery, 1995: 202).

A nursing curriculum based on the radical view of education, specifically a critical curriculum perspective, would certainly look very different from that to which most nursing schools are accustomed. Coming from a tradition of behavioural objectives and content-driven curricula, most nursing education institutions have not even begun to interrogate their own curricula and practices. A complete paradigm shift toward an understanding and an appreciation of the inextricable nature of health and disease in the socio-cultural, economic and political context, as well as an awareness of the fact that individual, societal and institutional responses to health and disease are largely a function of the context

Table 1.2 Advantages and disadvantages of the three types of curriculum approaches

Curriculum approaches	Advantages or strengths	Disadvantages or weaknesses
Content-based approach	Teacher has control over what is taught Content can be carefully chosen Much content can be covered in relatively little time It is easier than the other two types to organize	Few competencies might be mastered Independent learning is not fostered, since the curriculum is teacher-focused Teaching easily becomes irrelevant, since it takes much time and effort to change them Teaching easily becomes irrelevant, since there is no direct link with practice It may lead to over-teaching
Process-based approach	It teaches nursing in a way which is in harmony with the scientific approach of the discipline (problem-solving in partnership) It is a motivating way of teaching and learning It is student-centred Since knowledge is attained in context, it is remembered more easily It encourages personal development of the student Students learn how to learn, which promotes life-long learning	Changing to this kind of curriculum demands much time and preparation of the school and the teachers In large schools the small group teaching demands many teachers
Outcomes-based approach (technological pragmatism)	Allows for flexible trajectories of learning Ensures certain skills levels in graduates Increases motivation since relevance is immediately obvious Bridges the gap between vocational and academic education The curriculum usually allows for different pathways to the outcomes, and this allows for more individualization and contextualization Learning outcomes are clear, and evaluation is potentially more valid and reliable	It demands that both teachers and learners learn new ways of working If the curriculum is not planned to be coherent, with different modules connected systematically, learning can be fragmented Might become over-specialized, with broadening aspects of education neglected

Table 1.2 continued

Curriculum approaches	Advantages or strengths	Disadvantages or weaknesses
Outcomes-based approach (social reconstructionism)	Provides a broader understanding of health and disease Development of capacity for questioning and challenging of the status quo for and with the clients of nursing Broad definition of competence to ensure that the education of nurses does not become overly technocratic and behavioristic Potential for preparing a politically aware and conscientized nursing workforce to lead health sector reform	Potential to be more rhetoric than action with nurses perpetually living in a utopia Potential for action without thought resulting in revolutionary action rather than transformative action The bureaucratic and rigid nature of the healthcare settings might prove to be impenetrable by emancipatory ideals leading to pessimism and nihilism on the part of the nurses The extent of inequity and associated health status of the community might be too overwhelming for nurses and lead to feelings of despair and sense of futility in the face of large-scale inequities and their debilitating consequences in the lives of communities

Albanese and Mitchell, 1993; Wellard and Edwards, 1999 – excluding OBE as social reconstructionism.

in which nurses have to function are advocated. In the words of Varcoe (1997) 'A radical philosophy of education would seek to transform not only the relationship between teachers and students, but also the relationship between nurses and clients, and ultimately the health care system?' (1997: 198).

Instead of using objectives and/or content outlines as a starting point, the following questions should be used:

- What knowledge is currently taught in nursing schools?
- Whose knowledge is it?
- What role does such knowledge serve in legitimating and/or unsettling universal interpretations of health and disease – that is germ theory versus social, political and economic determinants of heath?
- In the context of the current forces shaping individual and population health, what knowledge and/or skills are important for nurses to know?
- What purpose should a nursing curriculum serve – helping clients and students adjust to their domestication or help them understand and act with a view to a transformed heathcare policy and system?

From the critical curriculum perspective, therefore, professional education, including nursing education, cannot be divorced from the social, political and economic contexts that shape it. A comparison of the three approaches to curriculum with regard to their advantages and disadvantages appears in Table 1.2.

Conclusion

Curriculum development in nursing education, has for a long time, whether knowingly or unknowingly, proceeded from some philosophical perspective. Examining the philosophical foundations from which the nursing education institution wishes to proceed and making these explicit to the learners and the public might bring some coherence into the educational practice of nursing education institutions. Admittedly, for the most part, none of these ideological views will be used in isolation, but clarifying beliefs about the purpose of nursing education, the range of views about knowledge and the roles of the teachers and learners in the educative process might serve as both starting points and criteria for monitoring one's practice against the institution's espoused philosophy of nursing education.

References

21st Century Schools (2004) *Designing a curriculum – Curriculum theory and critical pedagogy in the 21st century*. Online. Available at: http://www.21stcenturyschools.com/designing_a_curriculum.htm (accessed 12 March 2004).

Albanese, M. and Mitchell, S. (1993) Problem-based learning: a review of literature on its outcomes and implementation issues. *Academic Medicine*, **68**: 52–81.

Beyer, L. E. (1986) The reconstruction of knowledge and educational studies. *Journal of Education*, **168**: 113–135.

Bode, B. H. (1937) *Modern Education Theories*. New York: The MacMillan Company.

Cuffaro, H. K. (1994) *Experimenting with the World: John Dewey and Early Childhood Education*. New York: Teachers College Press.

Dewey, J. (1897, 1998) 'My pedagogic creed.' In L. A. Hickman, and T.M. Alexander (eds) *The Essential Dewey – Volume 1: Pragmatism, Education, Democracy*. Bloomington: Indiana University Press.

Dewey, J. (1916, 1961) *Democracy and Education*. New York: MacMillan.

Eisner, E. (1994) *The Educational Imagination: On the Design and Evaluation of School Programs*. New York: Macmillan College Publishing.

Ernest, P. (1991) *The Philosophy of Mathematics Education*. London: Farmer Press.

Freire, P. (1972) *Pedagogy of the Oppressed*. London: Penguin.

Freire, P. (1998) *Teachers as Cultural Workers: Letters to Those Who Dare to Teach*. Boulder, Colorado: Westview Press.

Gaudelli, W. (2002) U.S. kids don't know U.S. history: The NAEP study, perspectives, and presuppositions. *The Social Studies*, **93**: 197–201.

Giroux, H. (1988) *Schooling and the Struggle for Public Life: Critical Pedagogy in the Modern Age*. Minneapolis: Minnesota Press.

Gross, S. J., Shaw, K. M., and Shapiro, J. P. (2003) Deconstructing accountability through the lens of democratic philosophies. Online. Available at http://www.uiowa.edu/~jrel/spring03 (accessed on 12 March 2004).

Hearne, J.D. and Cowles, R.V. (2001) Curriculum development: a critique of philosophical differences. *Education*, 108(1): 53–56.

Hickman, L. A. (1998) Introduction. In L. A. Hickman (ed.) *Reading Dewey: Interpretations for a Postmodern Generation*. Bloomington: Indiana University Press.

Kilgour, D. (1995) Whither educational thinking? *Canadian Social Studies Magazine*, 30. Online. Available at http://www.david-kilgour.com (accessed on 12 March 2004).

Mason, M. (2000) Teachers as critical mediators of knowledge. *Journal of Philosophy of Education*, 34: 343–352.

Moore, R. (2000) For knowledge: tradition, progressivism and progress in education – reconstructing the curriculum debate. *Cambridge Journal of Education*, 30(1): 17–36.

Noddings, N. (1995) *Philosophy of Education*. Boulder, Colorado: Westview Press.

Novack, G. (1975). *Pragmatism versus Marxism: An Appraisal of John Dewey's Philosophy*. New York: Pathfinder.

Reed, D. F. and Davis, M. D. (1999) Social reconstruction for urban students. *The Clearing House*, 72: 291–294.

Slattery, P. (1995) *Curriculum Development in the Postmodern Era*. New York: Garland Publishing Inc.

Smeyers, P. (1995) Education and the educational project II: do we still care about it? *Journal of Philosophy of Education*, 29(3): 400–413.

Stern, B. S. and Riley, K. L. (2002) Historical legacy: linking Harold Rugg and social reconstructionism to 'authenticity' in theory and practice. *Curriculum and Teaching Dialogue*, 4(2):113–121.

Tanner, D. and Tanner, L. N. (1995) *Curriculum Development: Theory into Practice*. New York: Macmillan.

Tyler, R.W. (1949) *Basic Principles of Curriculum and Instruction*. Chicago: The University of Chicago Press.

Varcoe, C. (1997) 'The revolution never ends: challenges of praxis for nursing education'. In S. E. Thorne and V. E. Hayes (eds) *Nursing Praxis: Knowledge and Action*. London: Sage.

Walker, J.C. (1995) Towards a contemporary philosophy of professional education. *Educational Philosophy and Theory*, 27(21): 76–97.

Wellard, R. and Edwards, H. (1999) Curriculum models for educating beginning practitioners. In J. Higgs and H. Edwards (eds) *Educating Beginning Practitioners, Challenges for Health Professional Education*. Oxford: Butterworth-Heinemann Medical.

Weltman, B. (2002) Praxis imperfect: John Goodland and the social reconstructionist tradition. *Educational Studies*, 34: 61–83.

Wiles, J. and Bondi, J. (1998) *Curriculum Development: A Guide to Practice*. Columbus, Ohio: Merrill.

Chapter 2

An overview of the process of curriculum development

Leana R Uys

Introduction

Developing a curriculum is a major task, which should be seen as an ongoing process, rather than a one-off event. It commences when the nursing education institution makes a decision to develop a new curriculum, but it is never really completed. Even when a new curriculum has been implemented, and the implementation and outcomes have been evaluated, the process does not stop. Adaptations are usually necessary, and the impact of these has to be evaluated, and so the process continues.

The variables in the process of curriculum development are legion. Some examples are listed below.

Triggers for change

In some cases the triggers for change are internal to the organization; staff feel dissatisfied, or new staff with new ideas join the group. In other cases, the triggers are external; the regulatory body makes new demands, or the health services request new skills or content.

New or old

When a new programme is being developed, which was not offered at an institution before, a totally new curriculum has to be developed. When an old curriculum already exists, but needs to be modified, one can either base the new one on the old one, or start afresh on a totally new curriculum.

Programme complexity

Most pre-registration programmes have a number of levels, usually defined in years, and involve many subjects and many fields within nursing. Some post-registration programmes, however, have only one level, and may involve only one specialty area in nursing.

There is no single development process that is always the most appropriate. There is a basic process, however, that can be adapted to local and national situations. This is usually called the rational approach, which is a systematic process that a group of curriculum developers completes step-by-step.

Curriculum terminology

There are many terms that are used in this field, that are defined differently by different authors and education institutions. Even the basic term 'curriculum' has many meanings, and the choice of a particular meaning will greatly affect the process of developing such a curriculum. We will use the word curriculum to refer to planned learning experiences offered in a single programme.

A school of nursing

This is a department within a university, or a college or any other higher education institution that controls and administers formal nursing and midwifery programmes. It may also refer to the total higher education institution, in the case of a single-discipline institution. The head of school is the person, usually a nurse, who is the executive director of the school. The title might be dean, principal, professor, but the job is to give academic and administrative leadership.

A programme

This is a coherent set of courses, leading to a certain degree, diploma or certificate. In a programme there might be both core (compulsory) and optional courses (electives) (Vroeijenstein, 1995).

A course

This is a building block of a programme, consisting of a time-limited component, usually over one term (3 months), one semester (6 months) or 1 year, and usually ending with a summative evaluation.

A subject or a discipline

This is a clearly identifiable area of knowledge that considers and reviews a specific set of phenomena from a particular perspective, often using unique research methods (Miller, 1987).

A module

This is a unit within a programme or a course, which can be examined separately (modular instruction) or at the end of the course. It is sometimes left to the student to decide the order in which the modules are taken.

A learning opportunity

This is a learning situation created by a nurse educator for a student to use to achieve a learning outcome.

For example:

A school:	School of Nursing, University of Thimbuktu
A programme:	Bachelor's Degree in Nursing (BN).
Subject:	Nursing
Course:	Fundamentals of Nursing, Medical-surgical Nursing
Module:	Promoting healthy nutrition for a three-generation family
Learning opportunity:	Students are exposed to the process of carrying out a nutritional assessment with a family

---

Pre-registration and post-registration programmes

Pre-registration programmes are those which non-nurses take to become nurses. Such programmes usually lead to registration with the regulatory body as a nurse or midwife, and are the entry-level programmes of the occupation of nursing and midwifery. Post-registration programmes are offered to people who are already nurses or midwives to equip them for a specialized field of practice.

A level

A programme can have only one level, or can be made up of a number of levels. A level is a period during which the subjects or courses taken are at a similar level of difficulty, for instance first year courses might all be introductory courses to different subjects. At the end of a level, a decision is usually made about the progression of the student, based on a comprehensive assessment of the student's performance. There might be coherence between courses taken on the same level, for instance, a programme might have a course on family sociology in level one, to support a health promotion course taken at the same time.

Courses from different levels might also build on one another, for instance, having fundamental nursing in level one, and medical-surgical nursing in level two.

The process of curriculum development

Curriculum development is the process of deciding what to teach and learn, along with the considerations needed to make such decisions. It includes aspects such as tasks, roles, expectations, resources, time and space, and the ordering of all these elements to create a curriculum plan or document (Behar, 1994). Curriculum development is institutionalized change, which means that it is sanctioned by the formal structures in the educational institution. It is usually aimed at improving the situation, and therefore includes some form of evaluation and is carefully documented or described (Behar, 1994).

The national process

Regulatory bodies for nursing or for higher education often develop a national curriculum for specific nursing programmes. This is an essential development for the following reasons:

- The minimum standards of nursing and midwifery education should be nationally determined to ensure safe care for the population.
- National guidelines also ensure good quality of education for learners, who invest their time and money in achieving a qualification.
- National guidelines ensure that movement of nurses and midwives inside the country is possible, since they have all achieved the same basic requirements.
- Such guidelines also ensure that the national health priorities are included in all nursing and midwifery education.
- National curriculum reviews can also contribute to improving quality on a national basis.
- Since registration of nurses and midwives usually takes place nationally, a national curriculum is essential to standardize the competence guaranteed by registration (Glatthorn, 2000).

This national curriculum should be developed by curriculum specialists and leaders, since such development may require major re-orientation in nursing education. The expertise that is needed on such a national curriculum committee is closely linked to the tasks of the committee, which are outlined in Table 2.1.

A curriculum expert has to have a deep understanding of traditional curriculum practice (what is currently being done), vision and values that drive both the traditional practitioners and those asking for change, reforms and reform movements in education and nursing, and lastly research that could inform curriculum decisions (Becher and Maclure, 1978).

Table 2.1 Tasks of a national curriculum committee

Task	Expertise
1. Find and develop curricula that are markedly more effective in helping students become competent to give high quality nursing care.	Curriculum experts, nursing education researchers
2. Gain a working agreement among stakeholders on curriculum initiatives.	Key opinion formers from service, education and politics (students, professional organizations, labour unions).
3. Implement curriculum initiatives in a widespread, authentic, lasting way.	Nurse educators from all implementation levels. Those preparing nurse-educators. Education authorities and managers.
4. Evaluate the outcomes and impact of the new curriculum guidelines on nursing education institutions, graduates and the health services.	Programme evaluation experts, implementors and health service personnel.

From the start of the process, the developers have to plan for involving the greater stakeholder groups through a process of targeted consultation. This might include consultative open meetings or meetings to which a purposive sample is invited, questionnaires sent to individuals or institutions, and draft publications sent out for feedback. The developers should also plan for disseminating the information as it becomes available, to prepare implementors for the final guidelines and timelines.

The people who develop the national curriculum or national curriculum guidelines are also responsible for making sure that local educational institutions have the resources to implement the guidelines. If the essential resources are not available, guidelines are unrealistic, and cannot be authentically implemented.

The institutional process

The institutional process is even more important. Even if a national curriculum is available, it has to be interpreted by nurse educators locally. The teaching/learning philosophy of the local institution, the characteristics of local students and many other factors make such local interpretation essential (Walker, 2003).

The institutional process should be driven by a formally elected and/or appointed committee, on which all major stakeholders are represented. These include:

- Nurse educators at all levels of the educational institution, to ensure deep understanding of the context of the teaching/learning and the new curriculum, and to support implementation.
- Current and past students, to ensure that their experience of the current teaching/learning is taken into account, and to obtain their support for implementation.
- Health service personnel, to get the input from the practice site of students and graduates, and to improve understanding of vision and goals.
- Community members, to ensure that the needs of the community are addressed, and their support for change obtained (Young, 1998).

Many others, such as curriculum experts, subject specialists, political leaders, representatives of the professional regulatory body, professional and labour organizations could also be included from time to time. The four major groups must be included as members of the Curriculum Committee more consistently.

Leadership should ideally come from the head of the school. Heads often find it difficult to make time for this activity, but there are important reasons to make the time for it.

- A quality curriculum is essential for achieving educational excellence. In a survey of more than 3000 studies of student achievement, the quality of the curriculum was found to be one of the ten factors influencing student achievement (Glatthorn, 2000).
- Heads who use an active, initiating style of leadership have been found to be most effective in ensuring implementation of a new curriculum (Glatthorn, 2000). This style is characterized by clear long-term goals, strong expectations of students and staff, a positive attitude to change locally and nationally, involving staff, but acting decisively.

The Curriculum Committee should not work in isolation, but have regular and frequent feedback meetings with the rest of the staff of the school. The input of all stakeholders should also be sought when applicable during the process of developing the curriculum, so that their input is built into the curriculum. Between meetings the stakeholders can be kept in touch with developments through sharing the minutes of meetings, or by producing a newsletter.

Steps in the process

In the prescriptive approach to curriculum development, the following steps are followed to develop a curriculum:

Step 1: Establish the context and foundations

A thorough situation analysis is done to establish what the programme should aim to do, and how it should do it. These decisions are made based on the context of the programme; what is expected of graduates, what the resource base of the programme is, both within and outside the school, who the students are who will enter the programme, in which systems the programme will function and how this will influence the programme. During this phase the beliefs and vision of those involved in the programme are also established, to form the foundations of the programme, often in the form of a mission statement and a conceptual framework.

Step 2: Formulate the outcomes or objectives

In professional education, it is always essential to identify what competency the graduates of a programme have to achieve. This is based on the role they will play in the health services.

Step 3: Select a curriculum model and develop a macro-curriculum

The curriculum model (content-, process- or outcomes-based) will determine the internal structure of the curriculum. It includes the choice of learning opportunities and content, as well as the organization of these elements.

Step 4: Develop the micro-curriculum

This micro-curriculum is the level at which actual teaching/learning takes place. It includes the outlines of all courses, specifics about learning opportunities and evaluation strategies.

Step 5: Plan for the evaluation of implementation and outcomes

Although this is written as step 5, it has to happen quite early in the process, so that the relevant data can be collected timeously. Implementation evaluation refers to monitoring to what extent the curriculum that is on paper is actually the one students experience. Outcome evaluation refers to monitoring the planned and unplanned results of the curriculum.

These steps cannot be seen as water-tight, since the group will probably find themselves going backward and forward between different steps. For instance, it is often when macro-curriculum decisions have to be made that the values of the group become clear. These can then be added to the mission statement. The steps will be further elaborated in the next few chapters.

The product

What does a comprehensive curriculum document consist of? There are many answers to this question, and regulatory bodies the world over have a range of requirements for such documents. Nevertheless, there are a number of documents that should be included if a description of the curriculum for a programme is to be given.

The situation analysis

This can be given as a separate component, or be incorporated into other components, such as a motivation or rationale for the programme, or a description of the setting and resources.

A philosophy or mission statement

One would expect that the teaching/learning philosophy of the school would be the same for all programmes, although the focus might shift somewhat from pre-registration to post-registration programmes. Such a philosophy can be in the form of a written statement, or a model or theoretical framework. It should be substantiated by the literature and the situation analysis.

Curriculum design

This is a brief description of the programme objectives, the type of curriculum used, and the organizational principles of the curriculum. There should always be a set of outcome statements, which describe the competence of the graduate that the programme aims to produce. Then there should be a clear indication of the type of curriculum chosen, how the curriculum is structured, and how learning opportunities are organized. The rationale for every curriculum decision should be given.

Macro-curriculum

Once the design has been described, the specific levels and content of each should be identified. If there are different levels in the curriculum, these should be indicated, and the progression outlined. The content of the curriculum (modules, subjects, courses), both core and optional, should be identified. For every course or module a short description should be written, to guide the developers of the micro-curriculum. In a nursing curriculum, the macro-curriculum also includes a placement plan, which outlines when and where students will be in the clinical setting, and how this fits in with their theoretical instruction.

Micro-curriculum

The micro-curriculum includes a course guide for each course, outlining the content, teaching/learning strategies and evaluation strategies. The course outlines may vary greatly depending on the type of curriculum. For instance, in a problem-based learning (PBL) curriculum, the paper problems and the facilitator guides will be part of the micro-curriculum.

Models of nursing education

Since the development of nursing as a modern health profession, three basic models of training can be identified. The model of nursing influences the curriculum extensively, since the aims of the different models vary greatly. For instance, secondary education prepares students more generally for adult life, assumes that the learner is a child, and addresses a wide range of subjects. Higher education assumes that the student is at least a young adult, with a range of life-learning skills, who is being prepared for a specific career choice.

The three dominant models are detailed below.

The Nightingale model

In this model the matron of the hospital is in charge of both nursing care and nursing education. In the time of Florence Nightingale, the matron reported to the hospital board, and not to the medical superintendent. Currently most schools using this model have the matron reporting to the hospital administrator. Students are usually accommodated in nurses' homes, and nurses working in the hospital are seen as part of the teaching team. This system is close to the apprenticeship system, and the hospital is often dependent on the nursing students as part of the workforce. Although the training of nurses is often postsecondary education, it does not fall within the ambit of the formal higher education system, but under the health system. This model still dominates in Anglophone countries in Africa.

The higher education model

In this model, which is the main model in Canada, the USA, the United Kingdom and Australia, nursing education is part of the higher education system. Nursing students are registered students at universities or equivalent higher education institutions, and these institutions arrange for clinical learning experiences either in affiliated or independent health services. Students are not part of the work-force of the hospitals, and hospital staff take very little responsibility for the learning of the students.

The secondary school model

In this model, the first level training of nurses is within the secondary school, where vocational training is done to prepare school leavers for a career. Nursing is taught within the secondary school system by secondary school teachers, with a variable level of clinical exposure. This is a model often found in Francophone African countries.

In all countries of the world these three models are adapted to fit the local situation, but one usually dominates. The model of nursing education will clearly have an enormous influence on the type of curriculum developed for the programme.

Conclusion

The development of a new curriculum is a powerful tool for change. Such developments can therefore be seen as an exciting time for those involved in them, but also as a demanding time, and one that might threaten people's comfort zones. Careful planning and strong leadership are demanded, and also enough time to do a thorough job. Trying to develop a new curriculum over a weekend, or having it done by a consultant or a small group in a corner, is not the way to get a quality curriculum. It is a learning-by-doing activity in which as many people as possible should be included.

Points for discussion

- Who should lead innovation in nursing education; the government, the nursing organization(s) or the nursing school? Why?
- How appropriate is the nursing education system in your country for the new millennium?

References

Becher, T. and Maclure, S. (1978) *The Politics of Curriculum Change*. London: Hutchinson & Co.

Behar, L .S .(1994) *The Knowledge Base of Curriculum. An Empirical Analysis*. Lanham, Maryland: University Press of America.

Glatthorn, A. A. (2000) *The Principal as Curriculum Leader. Shaping What is Taught & Tested*. Thousand Oaks, CA: Corwin Press, Inc.

Miller, A. H. (1987) *Course Design for University Lecturers*. London: Kogan Page.

Vroeijenstein, A. I. (1995) *Improvement and Accountability: Navigating Between Scylla and Charybdis. Guide for External Quality Assessment in Higher Education*. London: Jessica Kingsley Publishers.

Walker, D. F. (2003) *Fundamentals of Curriculum. Passion and Professionalism*, 2nd edn. Mahwah, NJ: Lawrence Erlbaum Ass.

Young, M. F. D. (1998) *The Curriculum of the Future*. London: Falmer Press.

Recommended reading

Overbay, J. D. and Aaltonen, P. M. (2001) A comparison of NLNAC and CCNE Accreditation. *Nursing Educator*, **26**(1): 17–22.

This is a useful article which gives information about the bodies (National League for Nursing and the Commission for Collegiate Nursing Education), the process of accreditation and the standards they use.

Sherman, D. W., Matzo, M. L., Panke, J., Grant, M. and Rhome, A. (2003) End-of-life nursing education consortium curriculum. An introduction to palliative care. *Nurse Educator*, **28**(3): 111–120.

Matzo, M. L., Sherman, D. W., Penn, B. and Ferrell, B. R. (2003) The end of life nursing education consortium (ELIVEC) experience. *Nurse Educator*, **28**(6); 266–270.

Together these two articles describe the process of curriculum development by a specific group of educators for a specific target group of students. They touch on many aspects of the process of curriculum development.

Chapter 3

Establishing the context and foundations

Leana R Uys

Introduction

No curriculum is developed in a vacuum. It is developed by a group of educators, for a group of students, in a specific school, set in a region of a specific country, with a health service and an education system that has its own unique characteristics. In order to develop a relevant, forward-looking and practical curriculum, the curriculum team needs to make a thorough study of the system in which the curriculum will be embedded.

Wragg (1997) gives three propositions that can be seen as the rationale for a situation analysis as the first step of the process of curriculum development. Firstly, education must incorporate a vision of the future, since education does not prepare students for today or yesterday, but for tomorrow. A situation analysis therefore has to try to predict what the future will demand of graduates. It has to look at trends and movements, and evaluate their strength and endurance. Secondly, there are escalating demands on people, both in terms of their chosen career, and in the wider world of living as a citizen in the 21st century. What was good enough for us might therefore not be good enough for current nursing students.

Thirdly, the learning of students must be inspired by several influences, without focusing narrowly on one aspect. The *how* of learning might be more important than *what* is learnt. For instance, future leaders might be shaped more by the attitudes, vision and inspiration they internalize during their education than by the content (facts) they were taught.

The challenge is therefore to study the context and the future in order to base the new curriculum on evidence and on best-practice. To do this, one should see the programme as an educational system, and use the systems approach to study the system.

Studying the context

Carrying out a situation analysis is not just a process of gathering information. While the group is studying the situation, certain decisions are usually already made, which become the guideline for later stages of the process. The situation analysis is also never really completed. The group often finds that decisions they make about the programme necessitate gathering further information not previously accessed, or the situation changes, and new facts come into play. Nevertheless, a thorough baseline situation analysis is essential.

What are the expectations people or groups have of the programme and to what extent are these being met?

In analysing a system, the expectations major stakeholders have, and the criteria for evaluation of the functioning of the system should be clearly described. In the case of an existing programme, which is being retooled, the extent to which the current programme meets expectations should be interrogated. In the case of a new programme, one should obtain the input of stakeholders with regard to what they would expect from such a programme.

With regard to nursing programmes, the following stakeholders are usually involved:

- Prospective students, and in the case of school-leavers, their parents.
- The health services who will employ the products of the programme.
- The health services in which clinical practica will be done during training.
- The education authorities, including the specific school or department in which the programme is offered, as well as the larger organization.
- The regulatory body for nursing, e.g. nursing councils or state boards.
- The community served by the educational institution and the health services.

All of these stakeholders usually have expectations of a programme, and the curriculum developers should find out what these are. If such expectations are ignored, the programme might disappoint the stakeholders, and this might lead to its failure.

An example: A neonatal nursing post-registration programme

A university nursing school is interested in launching a post-registration programme in neonatal nursing.

Provincial department of health: They want such a programme, but they insist that it be offered on a part-time basis, so that their nurses can take it without leaving their jobs. They also want it to be decentralized, so that nurses in rural areas can access the programme easily.

Prospective students: The nurses working in neonatal intensive care units (ICUs) are very interested in such a programme, but they want it to be at a Diploma level, since most of them do not have a B-degree, and could not access a Masters programme.

University: The university would prefer the programme to be at a Masters level, since this carries a higher government subsidy, and there is not much difference in the teaching input costs.

Hospitals in the area: Some want a neonatal ICU nurse, while others want a more generic ICU nurse. These administrators feel that preparing super-specialists, such as neonatal ICU nurses in a time of serious staff shortages, makes staffing more difficult.

Conclusions

Offer a part-time Diploma programme in neonatal ICU, with some modules also accessible to students registered for the general ICU programme.

What are the environmental influences on the program?

The environment refers to those influences from outside the system over which the system has little or no control. Nursing education forms part of at least four larger systems: the health system, the education system, the regulatory system and the societal system. The school has little control over the influence of these systems, and has to make sure that the impact is described and analysed. This does not only refer to the current situation, but also to trends that might indicate where the future lies.

The following list of questions could guide curriculum developers in analysing the environmental factors impacting on the programme they design.

Health system

1. Where does the prospective graduate fit into the health system?

   - Primary, secondary or tertiary service
   - Existing role or developing role.

2. What is the structure and function of the health system where the graduate will work?

Educational system

1. What is the educational philosophy and mission of the institution?
2. What are the current educational debates and developments in the profession, in the country and internationally?
3. What are the current debates in nursing education, nationally and internationally?
4. With what competence does the student enter the programme? From school education or previous professional education?
5. Has the school got competition in this field? Would it need to compete for students and resources?
6. What are the quality standards that impact on the development of this programme?
7. How is the system controlled? Which bodies have to approve the new programme? How much input has the school got on these bodies?
8. Does the school control its own resources?

Professional system

1. What regulations from the nursing regulatory body address this programme and what are the implications?
2. What are the new trends in the area of nursing covered by this programme?
3. What are the ethical issues to be addressed in this field?
4. What are the current debates in nursing which impact on this programme?

Societal system

1. Who are the health service users, in terms of language, culture, education, age and socio-economic indicators?
2. What are their health indicators, especially the ones indicative of the area of practice the programme prepares nurses for?
3. What are the presenting health problems of the consumers?
4. What is the influence of globalization on this programme? Should it ensure compliance with international standards?

The influences on the programme should be summarized in terms of their implications for the programme. For instance, the influence of different factors can be annotated to show in which part of the curriculum their influence is greatest.

For example: Excerpt from the situation analysis of a specialist qualification in paediatric nursing

Nursing council requirements:

The nursing regulatory body prescribes the content of this programme by indicating the subject names and number of hours of each that have to be included. However, it also stipulates that these are only guidelines, and schools can motivate for different combinations.

Note: Refer to rules only when doing macro-curriculum (choosing content).

Which resources can the programme access?

All resources that the school can access, either because it controls them (such as teaching staff) or because they can negotiate their use (such as clinical facilities) should be carefully analysed. A well-planned curriculum makes optimal use of all resources, and often uses resources in unique ways or combinations.

The following resources need to be analysed.

Teaching staff

1. Are there enough teachers for the new programme?
2. How appropriate are their academic and professional qualifications for the programme?
3. Do they have the competence in the nursing field and the educational approach considered for the programme?
4. How adequate is their support, e.g. office space, support staff?

Teaching resources

1. Are there enough classrooms of the correct type (e.g. seminar rooms for PBL teaching, lecture theatres for content-based curricula) to accommodate the programme?

2.   Is the library adequately equipped with regard to the content of the new programme?
3.   Is equipment such as computers, facsimile machines, photostating machines, telephones, overhead projectors, video players available and in good order?

Prospective students

1.   How many students need to be registered per annum to make the programme both academically and financially viable?
2.   How large is the pool from which students will be recruited?
3.   Are they financially able to register for the programme?
4.   Would employers be interested in sponsoring students for this programme?
5.   What is the level of interest in the programme from potential students?

Clinical facilities

1.   Are appropriate health facilities available for clinical placement of students for this programme?
2.   What is the quality of the physical facilities, the human resources and the service in these health services?
3.   What is the quantity of services – would it allow for sufficient learning to take place?
4.   Are these services positive about having the students placed there?

In describing the resources, it is useful to compare them with those of other schools or other programmes. This allows for strengths and weaknesses to be highlighted, and promotes effective planning. It is also useful to have people from other disciplines or institutions read the resource analysis, since they often look at things differently, and might bring useful perspectives to bear on the analysis.

Once the resources have been analysed, it is possible to make a decision about their adequacy, and plan to address gaps that exist. For instance, staff might need to be prepared for a new teaching approach, or additional library resources might have to be budgeted for. In many schools a major new development might demand external funding, and this takes time to access. It is therefore important that the situation analysis be done early in the process, and actions initiated to address specific needs.

An example: Reshaping the B Pharmacy degree at the University of the Western Cape (Butler and Ensor, 1994).

The external facilitator (Ensor) and the Head of the School of Pharmacy met to discuss the views of the Head with regard to the need for change and the role of the external facilitator.

A workshop was then held with all members of the school to discuss the process of developing a new curriculum, and the perceived obstacles. Three major issues were identified at this workshop: the balance between departments involved in the degree programme, the division among the four subject areas, and the staff–student ratio.

Interviews were then done with employers and students (current and past) to evaluate the current programme and get their input on possible changes. Employers pointed out the changing role of pharmacists, while students criticized the irrelevance of large content areas of the curriculum, as well as the practical placements.

A second workshop was held, at which the participants studied the data gathered, and developed a profile of a 'complete graduate'. Based on this consensus, a working group was elected to develop a macro- and a micro-curriculum.

The group introduced a new component to the curriculum in the form of a clinical placement programme from the second to the final (fourth) year. They then developed the course content around this practical core. This central change addressed all the issues identified by the school, students and employers, and introduced a whole new way of training pharmacists.

Formulating curriculum foundations

A curriculum is never built on external and internal 'facts' only. The belief systems and values of the teachers and the system (educational and socio-political) in which they function, have to be factored in. This is done by way of developing a mission statement.

A mission statement is a relatively permanent and broad statement of the objectives of an organization, distinguishing it from other similar organizations and illustrating the main reason(s) for its existence (Pearce and David, 1987). This concept originated in the business world, but has been adopted in many fields, such as education. A mission statement is usually based on a thorough situation analysis, which incorporates the needs of society. It also articulates the values of the organization – their beliefs about what is important, and what they and their services are all about. A vision statement is closely aligned to a mission statement, but is usually a one-line statement that summarizes the core of the identity of the organization.

In education, a school might have a well-formulated mission statement, which covers all the programmes they offer. Such a mission statement has the function of creating a sense of community in a large organization, and unites the staff in a chosen direction. If such a mission statement does not exist, the team working on a curriculum could formulate a mission statement for their particular programme.

The following elements might be included in a mission statement:

- historical background
- educational philosophy and objectives
- orientation regarding the function of the institution
- obligations towards interest groups (Glatthorn, 2000; Strydom, 1989)

Example: Mission statement of a University Nursing School

Vision statement: Access to excellence in education towards service and research.

Mission statement:
The School of Nursing at the University of Kilima believes that under-graduate and post-graduate education for nurses should be available as widely as possible to enhance the ability of the nursing and midwifery profession to address the development needs of individual professionals and the health needs of the country.

Nursing and midwifery are two caring professions essential to the healthcare system of Africa. Nursing is caring for the health of an individual, a group or a community within a professional partnership relationship.

It further believes in providing innovative, process- and outcomes-based education, which develops the individual student into a self-directed, life-long learner, and links its graduates to an active academic network for life.

To ensure excellence in its programmes, it is essential to ensure that educators have intimate contact and collaboration with all types of health services, maximal academic development and active research involvement. Educators can only prepare nurse leaders and health leaders if they are themselves leaders in education, professional development, service delivery and research.

Historical background:
This school was established in the 1970s when it was realized that nursing education internationally was moving increasingly into universities, and that the nurses of this country were excluded from this development owing to limited access to under-graduate, bridging and post-graduate education. From the beginning it endeavoured to make university education accessible through distance, part-time and multi-media educational methods, while ensuring quality through the development of its teachers, and the continual evaluation and redesign of its programmes.

Included in the mission statement is usually a brief reference to the educational philosophy of the school, as well as the nature of nursing. What the teachers believe about the nature of knowledge, of teaching and of learning, needs to be identified and made explicit. This philosophical statement should be in line with the larger system in which the school is situated, and it should be reflected consistently in the curriculum.

The well-known Henderson definition of nursing says that nursing is assisting the individual, sick or well, in the performance of those activities contributing to health or its recovery (or to peaceful death) that she/he would perform unaided if she/he had the necessary strength, will or knowledge (Henderson, 1966). But this definition does not give adequate depth and clarity for curriculum decisions. For these reasons it is necessary that the group choose a nursing model or develop their own theoretical framework to describe what nursing is and is not. Without this clarity it will be difficult to make choices with regard to what to teach, how to teach it and where to teach it.

Glatthorn (2000, pp. 48–9) suggests the following process for developing a vision:

1. Get the stakeholders together, and explain the concept of a vision-statement, its use and the process of developing such a statement, to the group. Share the outcome of the situation analysis with them, so that they are fully informed about the current situation. If the group is large, it can then be divided into smaller groups of six to eight each for the next three steps.
2. Ask each individual to write a statement to complete the following sentence by adding between five to ten adjectives describing the essence of his/her vision, without any discussion with others:
    'The School of Nursing at X is . . . .'
    'The nursing programme X is . . . .'
    Each person then expands on the words in a few sentences.

3. Individuals now share their descriptive words (adjectives), and they are put onto the board. When all the words are there, clarification is sought about unclear ideas.
4. Each person then gets 3 minutes to advocate their adjectives, after which voting takes place. Each person has 15 points to allocate to the words on the board, to indicate which best represent the vision she/he has for the school or programme.
5. The group then discusses further the list with the most points, to make sure they adequately represent their shared vision, and to decide where the cut-off point is, that is, which concepts are in, and which are out.

From these words a draft vision statement is created, which is discussed more widely by all constituencies, before it is accepted. It will remain a document in process, which should be reviewed and adapted regularly.

It is not essential to develop a mission statement before anything else can be done. It may develop gradually as the group works on a new curriculum or a new programme. Once, developed, it should be used as a litmus test for all key aspects of the curriculum development process.

Conclusion

The curriculum committee should involve the larger stakeholder groups extensively in the process of analysing the context and establishing the foundations of the curriculum. Without such consultation, the information will not be complete, and the mission statement will not be valid. Even if such consultation has been continuous, the final draft should be presented for discussion and approval.

The product of this stage of the document is a thorough situation analysis, which not only describes the expectations, environmental influences and resources, but also makes a set of conclusions identifying strengths and weaknesses. It also includes a complete mission statement. These documents should form the basis of further curriculum planning, and should not be seen as a completed task, with the documents filed under 'done'.

Points for discussion

1. To what extent should a programme be shaped for local situation? Would this not lead to qualified nurses being unable to function in other settings?
2. How can the differences of philosophical beliefs of teachers in the same school be handled during the process of curriculum development?

References

Butler, N. and Ensor, P. (1994) Developing community-oriented pharmacy education: Reshaping the B Pharm degree at the University of the Western Cape. In: Walker, M. (ed) *Curriculum Development: Issues and Cases. AD Dialogues* 2. University of the Western Cape: Academic Development Centre.

Glatthorn, A.A. (2000) *The Principal as Curriculum Leader. Shaping What is Taught & Tested*. Thousand Oaks: Corwin Press, Inc. Sage.

Henderson, V. (1966) *The Nature of Nursing*. New York: The Macmillan Co.

Pearce, J. A. and David, F. (1987) Corporate mission statements: The bottom line. *Academy of Management Executive*, 1(2): 109–116.

Strydom, A. H. (1989) *Mission Formulation and Reformulation at Tertiary Education Institutions*. Bureau for University Education, University of Orange Free State: Bloemfontein.

Wragg, E. C. (1997) *The Cubic Curriculum*. New York: Routledge.

Recommended reading

Tiwari, A. (2002) Stakeholder involvement in curriculum planning. Responding to health care reforms. *Nurse Educator*, 27(6): 265–270.

This article describes how 70 people from nine different stakeholder groups were involved in the situation analysis of a school in Hong Kong, when they changed the curriculum of their masters programme.

Reutter, L. and Williamson, D. L. (2000) Advocating health public policy. Implications for Baccalaureate nursing education. *Journal of Nursing Education*, 39(1): 21–26.

This article illustrates the relationship between content and learning experiences.

King, M.S., Smith, P. L. and Glen, L. L. (2003) Entry-level competencies needed by BSNs in acute health care agencies in Tennessee in the next 10 years. *Journal of Nursing Education*, 42(4): 179–181.

This is a research article describing a survey done in an acute care setting, asking practitioners to rate 24 competencies in order to develop a relevant curriculum.

Chapter 4

Developing a macro-curriculum

Leana R Uys

Introduction

Having done a thorough situation analysis, the Curriculum Committee is now ready to proceed with the development of the curriculum itself. Some decisions will already have been made, or will at least have been discussed during the interpretation of the data collected during the situation analysis.

The macro-curriculum refers to the overall design or blueprint of the programme, and is done by a Curriculum Committee. In contrast, the micro-curriculum refers to the course outlines and unit plans, which are usually developed by the individual teacher. The components of the macro-curriculum are:

- programme outcomes
- the content guidelines and teaching approach
- scheduling of teaching/learning over the programme period.

In some countries, the modular curriculum has become popular over the last few decades in higher education institutions. Modular curricula involve the division of the programme into limited units or modules of learning which are then assessed at the end of that unit, with the student building up a qualification through an accumulation of credits (Jenkins and Walker, 1994). Although the basic approach of attaching a certain number of academic credits to courses in a programme is often used, professional programmes are usually more structured, with the overall coherence and the systematic development of professional competence central to its development.

Introduction to outcomes

Since nursing is a professional discipline, it is suggested that a competency approach be used to formulate the programme outcomes of nursing programmes. Competence is the ability to deliver a specified professional service.

This service refers to the total role functioning of the professional, and incorporates a number of units of competence (Ashworth and Saxton, 1990). A unit of competence (a competency) is a relatively self-contained achievement and should as far as possible be complete. It describes the outcome expectations of a particular work role and acts as a benchmark against which individual performance is judged.

Although there are curriculum approaches that are not based on outcomes, for instance content- and process-based curricula, it is impossible to conceive a curriculum, in a profession such as nursing, which does not identify the competencies of a graduate.

Outcomes have two main functions. Firstly, outcomes assist the developers of the curriculum and the teachers to make more effective decisions. Given clear outcomes, appropriate content and learning experiences can be chosen and evaluation strategies can be tailored to the expected competence. The process of deliberating about different outcomes, and choosing the final set, may be as important as the final decision, since it clarifies issues and directions for the team. The second function of outcomes is to orient the student to the expectations of the programme. This may not only decrease anxiety, but also improve the learning of the student by acting as an advanced organizer of learning inputs received.

Types of outcomes

Outcomes are used at different levels of a curriculum (Figure 4.1).

Terminal or programme outcomes

Terminal or programme outcomes describe the general destination of the students in a specific programme to which all teaching/learning is directed. It is the operationalization of the situation analysis and the philosophy of the school or the programme. It is also sometimes described as the 'characteristics of graduates'. The statements are comprehensive, but also clear and attainable.

Level outcomes

Level outcomes describe which goals should be achieved earlier, and which should be achieved later in the programme. These are used to organize the content and learning experiences of a multi-level programme. Level outcomes cut across and incorporate all the courses taken during that level of study.

Course outcomes

Course outcomes are formulated for a specific course and indicate what the goals of that specific course are. Course outcomes in nursing may draw on

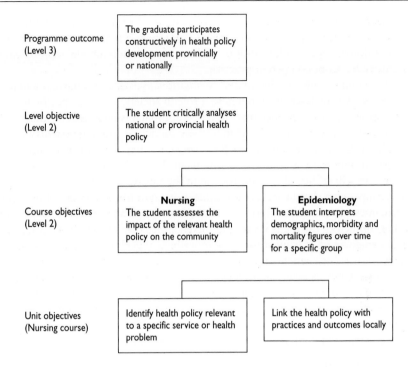

Figure 4.1 An example of different types of outcomes

knowledge gained from basic biomedical and social sciences, but are directed at nursing competence.

Unit outcomes

Unit outcomes are the most specific type of objectives, and refer to learning within a course. Unit outcomes are often formulated to be measurable.

All outcomes in a programme should be convergent, working in the same direction, and form a harmonious whole. There should not be contradictions or conflicts between outcomes.

Criteria for stating outcomes as competencies

The critical elements in understanding competency are:

- The focus is on *what the person can do* – on performance (Burke, 1995). Performance and competence are holistic concepts, which include knowledge, understanding, skill and attitudes. Competence demands that all these are appropriately combined into effective functioning. Skill without knowledge, understanding and the foundation of the appropriate attitude, is not competent practice.

- The competencies are *broad and occupationally based*, not narrow and job based. A role description refers to a role in society, not to a specific job in a specific setting. An occupation-based approach is intended for all nurses of a specific category or level in a whole service or region or country.
- Competence makes *provision for change*, so that the student is not prepared only to do the job at this moment, but to learn and adapt, so that she/he will still be able to do the job in the future.
- Competence should *focus on output*, not input (Burke, 1995). When one defines competence in terms of skills, knowledge and attitudes (explicitly or implicitly), the focus is on input. Even a focus on specific tasks is seen as input-focused. It is most useful to describe competence in terms of holistic work roles or elements of roles.
- Competence is something that is *inferred from performance*, and not directly observed. One usually observes only a segment of a person's functioning in the role. The assessment of competence is therefore dependent on more than one reliable and valid measure. The integrated approach to assessment of competence however, focuses on holistic assessment, as far as possible in the real situation.

The South African Qualification Authority (SAQA, 2000) presented a useful format for comprehensive outcome statements:

- a title which identifies the competence
- an element of competence (function), which is a significant role component
- performance criteria: quality statements that stipulate how well a task should be done
- range statements, which describe the context in which competence should be demonstrated.

This comprehensive statement is not appropriate at all levels of the curriculum, since outcomes become more detailed as the curriculum moves from macro- to micro-development. Programme outcomes will therefore usually have only the element of competence or the function, while at course outline level all four components will be present.

An example of a comprehensive outcomes statement is:

- Title: nursing assessment
- Competence: carries out a comprehensive and systematic nursing assessment.
- Performance criteria:
  - Communicates in a culturally sensitive manner
  - Obtains all relevant data accurately
  - Records all significant data systematically and clearly
  - Adjusts procedures to age and gender of patient.
- Range statement: in clinical and home settings, should include individuals and families.

Formulating programme outcomes

Programme outcomes are derived from the roles for which the students are being prepared. According to Mitchell's 1987 model, a work role consists of four components illustrated in Figure 4.2 (Burke, 1995).

- Task or technical competencies have to do with the core business of the role. They are routine, sequential, procedural, predictable and have tangible outcomes.
- Contingency management competencies have to do with managing breakdowns in routines, procedures and sequences.
- Task management competencies have to do with the management of tasks to achieve the overall job function. They have to do with prioritizing, planning and adapting.

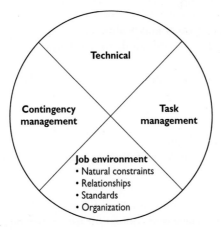

Figure 4.2 Components of work competency

- Role environment competencies enable the job holder to manage the natural constraints under which she/he works, working relationships, standards applied to the job, and the organization in which the job is performed.

The following criteria seem relevant to programme outcome statements:

- The competencies should be sufficiently broad to apply internationally or nationally.
- They should at the same time be specific enough to provide guidance in decision-making.
- The competencies should be fundamental to practice, and not peripheral.
- They should be relevant to practice.
- All occupational roles should be reflected.

Two examples of role statements and associated competencies:

A nurse who has just completed a pre-registration programme in nursing, should be competent to fulfil the role of a general nurse in the country in which she/he was educated. The registering body in the country will register her/him as a 'general nurse'.

This role might include the following competency (only one from the total list):

1. Provide nursing care to individuals with acute illness.
   1.1 Maintain nutritional and hydration status of patient.
   1.2 Maintain physical and psychological comfort.
   1.3 Prevent potential complications of the illness, the treatment and/or bedrest.
   1.4 Identify and manage complications.
   1.5 Promote recovery and healing
   1.6 Prepare patient and family for discharge.

A nurse who has just completed a specialist nephrology nursing programme should be competent to fulfil the role of clinical nurse expert in the country where she/he was educated. The National Association for Nephrology Nurses might put her/his name on their register as a nephrology nurse specialist.

This role might include the following competency (only one from the total list):

1. Provide dialysis for individuals with kidney failure.
   1.1 Assess the client and context for use of peritoneal dialysis.

1.2 Educate patient and family on implications of dialysis, the use of apparatus and the procedure of peritoneal dialysis and of haemodialysis.

1.3 Assess the cultural beliefs and values of the patient and family with regard to blood and transfusions.

1.4 Put patient on haemodialysis.

1.5 Identify problems with any type of dialysis and manage these.

The process of deriving programme outcomes in the form of competencies

Statements of competence should be derived from an analysis of functions within the area of competence to which it relates. This process is called a functional analysis, and it results in a functional map.

Step one: Define the role

Formulate the key purpose of the category or level of nurse viewed in very broad terms (Burke, 1995). Having done the situation analysis, and formulated the philosophy, it should be possible for the Curriculum Committee to write a role statement that makes clear what is expected from this group, as distinct from other groups of nurses or health workers. This process often begins with a long list of 'functions' or 'tasks' which are produced when a group is asked 'What should this person do, or what should this person be prepared for?' The Committee then has to integrate this list into a succinct role statement, which covers the essentials without going into detail. In such a role statement, the component roles should be clearly identified. While there is only one role statement an occupational group usually has more than one role component, for instance, nurses usually have a clinical role, a management role and a teaching role.

For example, a role statement for an advanced practice psychiatric nurse might be: An advanced practice psychiatric nurse (APPN) manages complex clinical cases, acts as consultant to other team members, and plans, implements and evaluates mental health programmes in institutions, communities and health districts. This role description has three components – clinician, consultant and programme manager. It distinguishes this practitioner from a first level psychiatric nurse, and is sufficiently broad to encompass the whole sub-group.

Step two: Develop an occupational map

Break this role statement into smaller components through a process of progressive desegregation, without losing sight of the key focus, and develop an occupational map. An occupational map identifies the role components of the group of nurses being prepared by the programme, and for each role component, the map describes the competencies that make up the role.

In the example in Table 4.1, the role of the APPN is segregated into the three main sub-roles, and one of them (3. Programme management) is then defined in terms of six competencies.

Table 4.1 The process of developing an occupational map with examples from the advanced practice psychiatric nurse (APPN)

Task one	*Decide on the desegregation (organizational) rules*
Explanation	This refers to the conceptualization of the key purpose in order to subdivide the role: will stages be used (e.g. the nursing process) or will components be used (e.g. primary, secondary and tertiary prevention) or will a combination be used
Example from APPN	The role components will be used. The role components of advanced practice psychiatric nurse include: 1. Managing complex cases 2. Acting as consultant 3. Programme management
Task two	*Formulate the first level of competency statements*
Explanation	For each of the role components, write a competency statement. In an occupational map the competency statement usually does not include performance criteria or range statements. This comes later in the process
Example from APPN	Using only role 3 above: 3. Programme management 　3.1 Evaluate the current programme in a specific setting or for a specific group 　3.2 Initiate change in an appropriate manner 　3.3 Plan a programme adjustment or revision with key stakeholders 　3.4 Build evaluation mechanisms into planning 　3.5 Implement planned change, and monitor effects 　3.6 Evaluate implementation and outcomes of the programme
Task 3	*Ensure that the list is complete*
Explanation	Check whether the role of the nurse is covered comprehensively by the role statements
Example from APPN	When checking the programme management list, no task management competencies were found Add: **7. Fit the programme change into the ongoing activities of the setting**

Step three: Ensure that the list is complete

This can be done by reviewing the literature, observing practitioners in real situations performing their roles, and discussing the occupational map with clients, practitioners, managers and educators (Fey and Miltner, 2000). The list should also be checked against the four aspects of job competence outlined by Mitchell (in Burke, 1995).

There are two common problems educators commonly voice when working with competencies. Firstly, educators often want to address knowledge, attitudes and skills separately as competencies, and secondly they doubt the possibility of adequately addressing high-level cognitive or attitudinal content in competency statements. With regard to the first problem, there is an approach that sees knowledge and attitudes as legitimate outcomes, in other words, that will accept competencies which refer only to knowledge or attitudes. This is not recommended, however, since it goes against the principle of integration of cognitive, attitudinal and psychomotor aspects into comprehensive competencies. It also goes against the principle of using a job focus in developing programme outcomes, that is, focusing on the job for which the programme is preparing the graduates. The second problem should be addressed by the correct understanding of competency. Knowledge, understanding and skills are implied by competencies and can be seen to be embedded within them, but competencies do not directly specify these elements (Burke, 1995). The level of knowledge underpinning a competency should be indicated by stipulating the performance criteria and range statements. Values need to be transformed from highly interpretative terms referring to some assumed internal state of the individual ('She values . . .' or 'He believes . . .') into something more concrete ('She treats equally . . .' or 'He involves clients . . .'). This transformation involves asking what the consequences are of having the assumed value or belief. The values of the profession should be clearly reflected in the role statement, and also in the individual performance criteria.

Selection and organization of content

Having formulated the programme outcomes, the next step is to choose the programme content and learning experiences, and decide on the organization of these. Content refers to the facts, concepts, theories, principles, laws, skills and attitudes students have to learn, while learning experiences refer to the ways in which the student engages with the content. The selection of content and learning experiences cannot really be distinguished from the organization of the curriculum. If the content is chosen in terms of subjects, the organization will be in terms of subjects. If the content of a course is chosen based on a specific textbook, the organization of the course will probably be according to the chapters of the textbook.

The macro-curriculum is heavily influenced by the type of curriculum that is chosen by the team. There are basically three approaches to curriculum organization; organizing the curriculum by content, by outcomes or by process (see Chapter 1). It should be remembered that few curricula present as pure examples of one of these models. Most schools combine some elements of each of the three models in their approach to developing a curriculum. For instance, even though they might be using subjects to organize the content of the curriculum, they will most likely set course objectives, and evaluate students on certain skills or competencies. In a problem-based curriculum, teachers might include a list of competencies which have to be achieved during the course of studying a specific clinical problem, and might evaluate attainment of these at the end of the module.

Together with the philosophy, evaluation, the outcomes, content and learning experiences form the basic building blocks of the curriculum. Changing one of these should change all of them (see Figure 4.3).

Criteria for the selection of content

The selection of the content of the curriculum should be based on a process of investigation and consideration of alternatives. The following criteria should be kept in mind.

Validity and meaningfulness

To be valid and meaningful, the content should reflect current scientific thinking and evidence-based practice. It also means that the curriculum should focus on fundamental knowledge, rather than superficial or peripheral details. The more fundamental an idea is, the more widely it can be applied. This kind of learning is often referred to as 'principle' learning, as opposed to 'fact' learning.

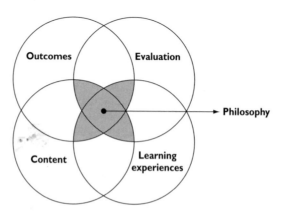

Figure 4.3 Elements determining content and organization

For example:

Principle: Increasing a person's understanding of a new situation decreases stress and increases coping.

Facts:
1. Orienting a patient who is newly admitted decreases anxiety.
2. Teaching a patient newly diagnosed with an illness about the illness prevents complications.
3. Involving the family and teaching them about the illness and care increases their coping.

Knowledge is more meaningful if it is introduced in a manner that communicates the spirit and method of the science at the same time. For instance, the method of philosophy is debate. Introducing philosophy in the form of debate therefore communicates content and method at the same time, and makes it more meaningful. If problem solving is seen as the basic process in nursing, then content offered in the form of problem solving is more meaningful than content offered as stories.

Relevance to the social context

A relevant curriculum is one that is built on the actual reality in which the graduate will practice. The real social, economic, occupational, judicial, political and geographic reality should have been explored during the situation analysis. These realities should now inform the decisions about curriculum content.

One of the newer curriculum models in the health professions is the community-based curriculum, advocated by the World Health Organization in the 1980s (1987). In this kind of curriculum the students are placed in community settings (as opposed to hospital settings) early in their educational programmes, and for a large proportion of their clinical experience. One of the major arguments for this kind of curriculum is that it makes the learning more relevant to the lives of clients and provides the students with richer learning experiences (see Chapter 11).

A few of the important realities of today's world are globalization, the fast pace of change, the development of technology, and early discharge, to name but a few. Unless a curriculum chooses content with these realities in mind, and equips students to deal with this world, it is not relevant. For instance, familiarity with modern technology such as computers, software programmes and internet use is not a luxury in a curriculum. It is essential to develop students into technologically literate professionals. Another example the models used in teaching nursing should enable students to work with families as caretakers in the light of the short hospitalization time of the average patient, and the high level of home care required.

A balance between breadth and depth

There is a continuous tension between knowing a little about everything, and not having an in-depth knowledge of important aspects, and knowing nothing about some things, but having mastery of the important aspects. No curriculum can escape the dilemma of making choices about what has to be included, and what should be left out.

There are many educators who do not feel comfortable if they have not 'covered everything' with students, and who feel very bad if a topic comes up in the clinical situation which they have not dealt with in the classroom. (See Chapter 1 for the basic assumption underpinning an essentialist view of knowledge.) This group will probably prefer to err on the side of superficially dealing with all topics, and will probably support a content-type curriculum. If the tendency to include everything is taken to extremes, it leads to a lack of depth, since covering large volumes of content in a short space of time leaves learners very little time to engage with the content.

Another group wants to make sure that students learn the essential and/or common material at the level of mastery, even though this might mean leaving many topics out altogether. This group tends to support process-type curricula, and believes that if the students have mastered the learning and problem-solving processes, they will be able to handle new topics independently. Alternatively, they might choose an outcomes-based curriculum, and believe that it is essential to ensure a competence in essential role components and not in 'head knowledge'. These approaches can be criticized as not covering the field broadly enough, or even not attaining adequate understanding (depth) of what is studied.

The ideal curriculum walks a fine line between too many topics without mastery and in-depth understanding, and too much depth with students being unable to cope with the range of problems confronting them in practice. The answers have to be found within the curriculum model chosen, and by including practitioners in the Curriculum Committee, who can assess breadth and depth in the light of practice experience. Finally, whatever choices are made, they have to be in line with the espoused philosophy of the nursing school.

Criteria for the organization of content

By definition a programme is a 'coherent set of courses' (see Chapter 2), and therefore the curriculum has to make clear how the programme is organized. The vertical relationships in a curriculum refer to how different levels of the programme relate to each other, while the horizontal relationships refer to how elements within the same level relate to each other.

The questions the committee has to address during this phase of the process include: What are the building blocks of the curriculum: modules, courses, subjects or a combination of all these? What is dealt with first (which subjects are offered in level one), and why? How does the programme progress to the final level? Are courses or modules seen as independent and interchangeable, or are they progressive, with some being prerequisites for others? How are the organizational decisions made; what are the principles of organization? To make sure that the curriculum is coherent, there should be clear organizing principles according to which the Curriculum Committee makes its curriculum decisions.

Principle of continuity

Continuity refers to the vertical repetition and elaboration of important elements of the curriculum. A concept or process is usually presented in a simple form, and then elaborated on in terms of complexity, breadth, depth and sophistication required from the student in its use. The concept is often not changed, but learning experiences in which it is used are selected to achieve greater elaboration.

To ensure continuity, curriculum strands are used. A curriculum strand is a repetitive idea or concept which appears throughout the curriculum and forms the framework for the choice of content and learning experiences. Two types of curriculum strands are usually used:

- Horizontal strands: These strands are introduced early in the programme, and applied in almost every learning experience during the programme. Examples are the nursing process, the health care system, and ethical principles.
- Vertical strands: These strands develop progressively over the different levels of the curriculum, so that the requirements from the learning experience and from the student change over time (NLN, 1974). Examples are given in Figure 4.4.

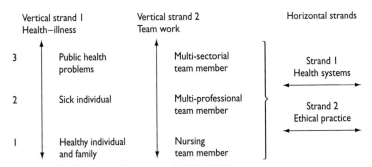

Figure 4.4 Curriculum strands in a three-year pre-registration nursing programme

Principle of order

Order refers to the sequencing of learning experiences and the presentation of concepts. A few examples of organizing principles are:

- simple to complex, e.g. teaching sociological concepts, before teaching sociological theories
- whole to parts, e.g. presenting a total case, and then looking at different aspects of it
- parts to whole, e.g. explaining how cells work, then tissues, and then organs
- chronological, e.g. teaching developmental psychology by starting with the development from baby to elderly person
- taxonomies, e.g. using Bloom's taxonomy of cognitive development to differentiate between what first year and second year students should be able to do
- health to illness, e.g. introducing students to healthy children and their development before teaching about the care of sick children.

To promote a logical coherence in the curriculum, the Curriculum Committee should make sure that course objectives support the level objectives, and that level objectives support the programme objectives.

An example of a horizontal strand in a pre-registration programme

Horizontal strand:	Team work.
Programme outcome:	The graduate works harmoniously and productively in all kinds of teams, ensuring that nursing input is maximized for the benefit of individuals, families and communities.
Level 3 outcome:	The graduate actively engages people and/or agencies from other sectors in identifying needs of communities, and maintains such relationships to the benefit of community health.
Level 2 outcomes:	The student interacts productively in multi-professional settings to promote good patient care. The student professionally articulates and illustrates the contribution of nursing in a multi-professional care setting.

Level 1 outcomes:	The student takes responsibility for work delegated to him/her by the nursing team leader. The student interacts productively with other nursing team members in nursing records, at team meetings and informally to promote good nursing care. The student promotes good team functioning through friendly, supportive and professional interpersonal relationships.

Principle of integration:

Integration refers to the horizontal relationships between learning experiences (courses, content, clinical placements) offered at the same time in a particular level. Integration can assist the student to see the greater whole of what is being learnt, instead of fragmented pieces. Integration of knowledge actually takes place in the student, but it can be facilitated by the way in which the curriculum is structured.

Integrated curricula based on conceptual frameworks of what nursing is, became popular in the 1970s. In many of these curricula the historic subjects such as physiology and psychology and nursing disappeared, and were integrated into 'Understanding children and caring for them' or 'The care of adults'. In many problem-based curricula the so-called 'basic medical sciences' and social sciences are also not taught separately, but are integrated into the problem scenarios with which the students work.

This type of integration is not essential to achieve horizontal coherence, but is only one approach to achieving a holistic view of knowledge. Other ways are to make sure that subjects taught at the same time support each other, that the timelines of subjects are similar, and that teachers consciously use the information from other subjects taught at the same time in their teaching. For instance, if the students are studying physiology while studying medical-surgical nursing, it would help if they deal with the cardiovascular system simultaneously in both subjects.

One way of promoting horizontal coherence is to use a nursing model or framework in the planning of the curriculum. A conceptual framework of nursing is a set of concepts which organizes the vast field of nursing in a set of meaningful units. This set of units can then be used as organizing principles for the curriculum, since it not only identifies what should be included in the programme, but also how these units relate to each other, and what the logical sequence is.

Developing course outline

Whatever model is used, the building blocks are almost always in different courses. For the macro-curriculum, each of these courses should be described briefly, in order to allow the reader to understand the curriculum. Such an outline should include at least the following.

Name of the course

In a content-based curriculum, educators are urged to use recognized names for academic disciplines, since this facilitates recognition by other educational institutions to which the student might apply in future. For instance, if a curriculum integrates physiology and pharmacology into a problem-based approach to nursing, a course might be called 'Understanding nursing of common ailments', and the description should then make clear that it is not purely a nursing course, but includes other sciences.

Place in the curriculum

It should be made clear where the course fits into the programme, both in terms of level and in terms of prerequisites. If the course is required for progression to the next level, this should be indicated. Which courses are compulsory and which are electives should also be indicated.

The description

This should indicate what content is covered in the course (concepts and/or processes), and how it is to be covered. This description should be detailed enough to allow the developers of the micro-curriculum to base their course decisions on the description. It should not be so detailed, however, as to leave the micro-developers no academic freedom.

The structuring of the clinical learning experience

The selection of the type and setting for clinical learning experiences forms part of the macro-curriculum. The level of clinical experience required of students during programmes differs greatly from country to country, often related to the requirements of the regulatory body, and the practice context.

A few factors influencing clinical placement are:

- In many developing countries, student nurses still form a major part of the workforce in hospitals, and this means that their clinical placement is often dictated by service needs rather than learning needs.

- In schools which are run by or affiliated to hospitals, there might be a reluctance to place students in other services, such as other hospitals, or in a community setting.
- Where resources for training are limited, educators might be forced to use clinical facilities in close proximity to each other, in order to limit cost for the school and for students. This might lead to an over-use of urban, better-resourced, more specialized types of health service.
- When educators working with pre-registration students are specialists in different nursing fields, they might tend to place students in such specialty areas, even though pre-registration programmes prepare generalists, and not specialists.
- Educationists often tend to place students in services rendering a high quality of care. If most of the services in a country are at this level or higher, that might be appropriate, but if most services are actually at a lower level, such a setting for training might not be appropriate. It might be an inadequate setting for training nurses to work in more challenging settings, where a higher level of professionalisms, interpersonal skills and innovation might be required. It might also tend to prepare nurses who do not want to accept the challenge of improving the quality of the national health service.
- In many countries regulatory bodies prescribe certain types and amounts of clinical learning experiences. This might be in the form of fields in nursing, and in number of hours of experience required. Schools are required to keep records of the clinical learning placements of students, since the professional registration of graduates is usually dependent on such information being provided by the training school.

The major questions the Curriculum Committee has to answer, are:

1. How much of the programme time will be spent in clinical learning?
2. How will the clinical learning experiences be spread across the total programme?
3. How will the clinical learning experiences be linked to the courses taken in different parts of the programme?

Classroom–clinical teaching/learning ratio

There are great variations between countries and between different types of nursing programmes with regard to the ratio between classroom and clinical teaching/learning. Large amounts of clinical learning experience are usually associated with apprentice-style education, while much less 'vocational' or 'practical' training is usually found in higher education settings.

To give a few examples: In a University School of Nursing in South Africa, students spend 3737 hours in clinical settings over a period of 4 years, while they accumulate 512 academic credits, which works out roughly to 1728 classroom hours. This means that the classroom:clinical ratio is about 1:2. In nursing colleges in South Africa, students spend 4880 hours in clinical settings over 4 years, and about 2160 hours in the classroom. The ratio in this school is therefore also about 1:2.

In a curriculum guide for pre-registration nursing and midwifery programmes in Africa, developed for the WHO African region in 2000, a classroom:clinical ratio of 1:3 or 1:4 was suggested (Uys, 2000). The large amount of clinical work was based on the premise that registered nurses in Africa often work with very little support, even soon after graduation. They therefore have to be competent to practice with minimal supervision on graduation. This might not be the expectation in all countries, and the expectations from the marketplace will influence the decisions made on this issue.

Structuring clinical learning experiences

There are basically three models of structuring clinical learning experiences (the 'block' system, the integrated system and the internship system) although there are many varieties within each of the basic types (see Table 4.2). For instance, the modular type curriculum can use a mini-block system for each module, or can use an integrated system for each module.

The block system

In this system the programme time is divided into 'blocks' which are dedicated to either classroom teaching or clinical placement. The advantage of this kind of arrangement is that students are relatively well prepared for the clinical areas in which they are to be placed, and the system makes scheduling easy for both the school and the clinical facility. Students are also in the clinical areas for continuous periods, which facilitates a good understanding of the role of the nurse in the particular clinical setting. They are also not subject to the stress of clinical placement when they have to prepare for tests and examinations. This system also allows for classroom teaching to be centralized, and clinical learning to be decentralized, since students move from the one setting to the other only at the beginning and end of each block.

In the best examples of the block system, the classroom teaching of a specific area of nursing precedes the clinical placement, there is some clinical exposure during the classroom block period so that the students can make immediate linkages, and there is some form of theoretical work during the clinical block period.

The possible problem with this approach is that classroom teaching blocks can become crammed with inputs, clinical learning can become 'work', without being linked to learning, and correlation of theory and practice might be difficult to achieve. Since the students are in the clinical area on a full-time basis during clinical blocks, there might also be the temptation for the service to move them from the allocated area to other areas, interfering with theory–practice correlation (Mellish and Brink, 1990).

The integrated system

In this system students are exposed to both classroom teaching and clinical learning every week. In pre-registration programmes the majority of student time is usually spent on the campus, with clinical placement taking place on one or more days per week. This system is often followed by university schools, since the programme has to fit the academic year. Students often take classes with other students, and therefore they have to fit in with the general academic calendar. In post-registration programmes, it is often the other way round, with students being in specialized clinical areas for most of the time, and having 'study days' for the classroom teaching.

In the best examples of this system, there is a close correlation between what the students are learning in the classroom and where they are placed in the

Table 4.2 Example: Stage one of a three-year programme in nursing

Block system	Integrated system

Jan to March: Anatomy
            Microbiology
            Psychology
Fundamental nursing
April to June: Clinical experience
(36 hours per week) in activities of
daily living in:
  Frail aged care centre,
  medical unit and
  health child clinics
August to October: Physiology
            Sociology
            Community health
            nursing
November to Dec: Health promotion
            project in communities
            Immunization clinics
	Semester one (15 weeks):
	Subjects: Anatomy
	            Microbiology
	            Psychology
	            Fundamental nursing
	Tuesday and Wednesday mornings:
	  Jan/Feb: Healthy baby clinics
	  March/April: Frail aged centre
	  May/June: Home-based care
	University Vacation period:
	Four weeks in medical/surgical units
	(36 hours per week).
	Semester two (15 weeks):
	Subjects: Physiology
	            Sociology
	            Community health nursing
	Tuesday and Thursday mornings:
	  July: Immunization and family planning
	            clinics
	  Aug/Sept: School health
	  Oct/Nov: Occupational health
	  University vacation period:
	  World AIDS day project (1 week)

Clinical learning experience hours: 810	Clinical learning experience hours: 496

health service. The same teachers teach both classroom and clinical, and clinical learning is used actively in the classroom setting and vice versa.

The advantages of this system are that it facilitates the integration of theory and practice, students have time to assimilate new inputs and apply them immediately, and lecturers are more involved in the clinical settings. The disadvantages are that it is much more difficult to do the scheduling, both at the academic and the clinical settings, and that students might have to deal with challenging emotional issues in the midst of dealing with academic demands. Students can also seldom pack in as many clinical hours as in the block system, since they have to travel to and from clinical placements. The restriction on teaching time may be seen as a disadvantage, but it also leads to a less packed teaching day, which is an advantage.

The internship system

This can be coupled with either of the previous systems, or can follow a programme which has very limited clinical learning experiences. It consists of a service-learning period following the formal 'academic' programme, and graduates usually have to complete this portion before they can register as professionals.

The best internship programmes include placing students in health settings where they can work with thoroughly prepared mentors, who are skilled and have the time to supervise and guide the internee. These include continued access of the internee to the learning resources of the school, both physical (libraries) and human (teachers), and a systematic feedback system to the student to ensure growth towards becoming a safe practitioner.

Theory–practice links

There are a number of ways in which the learning in the classroom can be linked to the experiential learning in health care settings:

- *Closeness in time*: If the student comes across an issue in the clinical setting very soon after having dealt with it in class, or vice versa, motivation for learning is increased. The student might also use the clinical case to remember the theory, or might use the clinical case to illustrate and understand the theory.
- *The same teacher*: If the teacher who teaches in the classroom, also follows the student into the clinical setting, there is a better chance of linking the one learning experience with the other. The teacher can refer the student confronted with a problem in the clinical setting to material dealt with in class, or remind him or her of a reading. Similarly, an example from the clinical area, experienced by some of the group, could be used to illustrate material in class.

- *Advanced directives*: When confronted by the wide range of stimuli inherent in the average clinical setting, students might not be able to identify what they should be concentrating on in order to learn. Although they might have been given a theoretical framework in the classroom, they could be provided with what Ausubel calls 'advance organizers' to help them to recognize the appropriate situation in which to apply the information in the practical setting (1960, p. 270). Such advance organizers could be checklists, lists of procedures they should master in a specific setting or objectives for their learning.
- *Using clinical material in the classroom:* Another possibility is to base the classroom learning on real experiences students have had in the healthcare settings. This can be done by using projects, case studies, service descriptions, and other forms of real data as the basis for classroom teaching/learning.

Many of these methods need to be built into the macro-curriculum from the start. For instance, if students are studying two or more fields of nursing at the same time, it is difficult and confusing to offer clinical experience in both close to the time of teaching. The Curriculum Committee might therefore want to modularize the curriculum to the extent that when the group is studying community health nursing, they are not at the same time studying medical surgical nursing, since one cannot place the student in such different settings at the same time. Similarly, if one wants the same teacher to follow students in the clinical area, one cannot use a block system which has the classroom teacher at a central point while students get their clinical learning experience in rural settings. The major decisions about linkage therefore have to be made during the macro-curriculum development stage.

Conclusion

The Curriculum Committee will do most of the work towards developing a macro-curriculum, based on the situation analysis done by the larger group. The work they have done should be presented to the larger group, however, with the opportunity for discussion, feedback and amendment. This presentation should include the total macro-curriculum; programme and level objectives, type of curriculum and curriculum strands, the content of each level, including the clinical placement (type, time and setting) and its linkage to classroom teaching.

The total macro-curriculum is usually the document which is presented to the institutional board for approval (e.g. University Senate) and also to the regulatory body (e.g. Nursing Council). For this presentation special formats might need to be used, according to the requirements of each body. The school should also keep a narrative description of the macro-curriculum which should be available to teachers who have to develop the micro-curriculum, to evaluators who monitor quality of the programme and to new staff members. As evaluation of and amendments to the curriculum are done over time, these should be added, so that a complete record of the curriculum and its implementation are kept for research and planning purposes.

Points for discussion

1. Jenkins and Walker (1994, p. 27) state that most recruiters of graduates would welcome a graduate who:
   - 'demonstrates intellectual ability (recognizes a need to know and knows how to find, interpret and use knowledge);
   - learns actively and independently (can identify his or her own learning styles and needs, and the means of meeting them);
   - has good self-management (can set targets, arrange priorities, deal with stress, work to deadlines, etc.);
   - is proficient in a range of transferable, general skills (information technology, problem-solving, teamwork, financial skills, numeracy, etc.);
   - has experience of working, understands something of the nature of working relationships, and has strategies for dealing with personal career decisions;
   - understands and can communicate personal abilities and achievement demonstrated while in university.'

Assess the degree to which the objectives in your own pre-registration nursing programme address these expectations.

References

Ashworth, P. and Saxton, J. (1990) On competence. *Journal of Further and Higher Education*, **14**: 3–25.

Ausubel, D. P. (1960) The use of advanced organizers in the learning and retention of meaningful verbal materials. *Journal of Educational Psychology* 51(5): 267–272.

Burke, J. (ed) (1995) *Outcomes, Learning and the Curriculum*. London: The Falmer Press.

Fey, M. K. and Miltner, R. S. (2000) A competency-based orientation program for new graduate nurses. *JONA*, **30**(3): 126–132.

Jenkins, A. and Walker, L. (eds) (1994) *Developing Student Capability Through Modular Courses*. London: Kogan Page.

Mellish, J. M. and Brink, H. (1990) *Teaching the Practice of Nursing*, 4th edn. Durban, South Africa: Butterworths.

National League for Nursing (1974) *The Process of Curriculum Development*. New York: NLN.

SAQA (2000) *The National Qualification Framework and the Standard Setting*. Waterkloof, South Africa: South African Qualifications Authority.

Uys, L. R. (2000) *Guidelines for a Basic Nursing and Midwifery Curriculum for the African Region of the World Health Organization*. Durban, South Africa: University of Natal.

WHO (1987) *Community-based Learning: An Approach to Medical Education*. WHO Technical Report Series No 746. Geneva: WHO.

Recommended Reading

Mahoney, M. A. A violence intervention and prevention program: The experience of Northeastern University (Massachusetts). In: Matteson, P. S. (ed) (2000) *Community-based Nursing Education*. New York: Springer Series on the Teaching of Nursing.

This chapter describes a community-based curriculum very well, and specifically a community-based health programme which has developed out of the school's involvement in the community. It gives a good idea of the problems and joys of such a programme.

Heinrich, C. R., Karner, K. J., Gaglione, B. H. and Lambert, L. J. (2002) Order out of chaos. The use of a matrix to validate curriculum integrity. *Nurse Educator*, 27(3): 136–140.

These authors use a matrix instead of curriculum strands, and give some examples of how this works.

Lanyk-Nhild, O. I., Crooks, D., Ellis, P. J., Ofosu, C., O'Mara, L. and Rideout, E. (2001) Self-directed learning: faculty and student perceptions. *Journal of Nursing Education*, 40(3): 116–123.

This is a research article, describing how the perceptions of faculty and students about self-directed learning change over time in a problem-based programme.

Chapter 5

Developing a micro-curriculum

Leana R Uys

Introduction

The development of the micro-curriculum is not usually done by the Curriculum Committee, but by small teams of teachers or individual teachers responsible for the teaching of that specific course. In some types of curriculum very detailed guidelines might be developed by the Curriculum Committee for the micro-curriculum. For instance, in a problem-based curriculum the format to be followed for the paper problems will be standardized across all levels and subjects. In some countries, where a national qualification framework is in place, and all qualifications have to be registered in a specific format, the basic outline of a course might be very clearly prescribed by the registering authority. In more traditional curricula there might be less uniformity, and teachers might have more leeway in developing their course outlines.

Wright (1994) pointed out that in each course there are three major influences on student development: the student, the course and the teacher. The course developers shape the course, and therefore their aims, their beliefs and their competence play a large part in the final outcome for the students and the teacher. The student, however, also plays a major role. Students enter a course with a particular conception of learning, variable levels of ability to cope with different learning tasks, and differing perceptions of their own abilities. The less prescriptive the course is in terms of content and structure, or the more options it gives students, the more students can shape the learning according to their own strengths and needs. The level of control the student is allowed depends on a number of factors, of which the course developers are the major one.

Advantages of a course description

The premise proposed in this book is that students should be empowered to be active learners by making the expectations very clear to them, whatever the curriculum model is. This means that when a student commences with a course, she/he should immediately be provided with a course guideline that describes the course comprehensively. This has a number of benefits.

- The student can plan his/her own learning programme, taking into account the expectations of all courses. Teachers sometimes act as though the student is only taking one course, and therefore feel that it is quite acceptable to spell out expectations and give tasks as the course progresses. This is not ideal, since the student has to juggle the demands of several courses, and cannot work systematically if the demands change from week to week.
- The student can estimate more clearly how much time he/she needs to schedule for the course. This allows them to make decisions about their other involvements, both academic and recreational.
- The student can access the resources for a specific task timeously, and not be caught short by an unexpected task.
- There is enough time for the student to seek clarification on tasks before the performance is expected. This prevents crises and calls over weekends and holidays.
- This approach ensures that the teacher does holistic course planning before teaching starts, and that it is not done in an ad hoc manner. As for the student, this allows the teacher to plan for more creative teaching approaches, and for the use of resources that need to be arranged.
- The criteria for evaluation are clear to students and teachers, and this clarity facilitates the achievement of objectives by students.
- Course outlines also facilitate a holistic perspective on knowledge, and facilitate integration of skills such as academic literacy, academic writing and numeracy over the total curriculum (Glatthorn, 2000).

Although one format is proposed in this chapter, there are many ways of approaching a course guideline. Essential, however, is that out-of-class tasks be set from the beginning, together with submission dates. It is also essential that the course and task objectives be given, together with evaluation strategies and criteria. A timeframe for the course is useful, as are the contact details of the teacher.

Course development

Based on the macro-curriculum, the small group of educators forming the course team now develops the course. This is a process of continuous interaction between the macro-curriculum and the knowledge base of the course team, during which a course is created. A course usually covers a full period of study, such as a block, quarter, semester or year.

The following might be useful steps in developing a course:

Step 1: Block in the course

Write the headings of a course outline, and fill in what you already know about the course, e.g. duration, placement, credits, etc.

Step 2: Formulate the course outcomes

Use the level or programme objectives to inform the choice of course objectives. Check with the curriculum strands, so that you pitch the course objectives at the appropriate level. Ask colleagues and students to read the objectives and check whether they are clear and specific enough.

Step 3: Divide the course into logical units of about equal weight

This can be done according to the time (e.g. one unit per week of the course), or by another form of logic (e.g. one unit for every activity of daily living in a fundamental nursing course).

Step 4: Develop the units

For each unit, decide what the essential tasks of the student will be (explaining, implementing, evaluating) and choose the appropriate content, teaching method, teaching/learning resources and assessment strategy. This step is much more time consuming if the curriculum is problem- or case-based, since in that case, it involves the development of the case materials (see Chapter 13). However, even in more traditional curricula the teacher needs to choose the teaching approach according to the expected learning outcomes. If one wants to teach students to teach patients, a demonstration is much more appropriate than a lecture. If one wants to teach students to interpret health indicator statistics, group work in class might be the best approach. In developing the course, a brief justification for the choice of content, and for the teaching approach is necessary, so that reviewers can understand the motivation.

Step 5: Select appropriate student assignments

Even in traditional courses, some form of self-directed learning is usually included. The overall weight of the course has to be taken into account when one decides how many assignments to put into the course. One should also consider whether they should all be individual assignments or whether some group assignments are more in line with the programme objectives, whether all should be presented in writing or whether some can be presented in the form of a tape recording or a demonstration, and whether the teacher should assess all of them or whether students can assess each other's projects for further learning. Once the assignments have been chosen, the assessment criteria have to be formulated. Again, a brief justification for the selection of the specific assignments should be included.

Step 6: Select appropriate teaching/learning resources

This might include videos, learning games, models, articles from journals, class-room visits by patients or their family members, field trips, and many more. Many of these resources will need some advance planning, and they may have to be acquired from outside the organization.

The primary teaching resources may be seen as being the teacher and the textbook, since obtaining additional resources is often expensive and time-consuming. One should thus use additional resources only when they are necessary. The following guidelines can be used to identify the need for additional resources:

- When an emotional response or attitudinal change is indicated, additional resources might be necessary. For instance, one can lecture to students about the need to talk to families of dying patients about the possibility of organ transplantation, but the impact of a visit from an articulate patient with renal failure might have a much more powerful effect.
- When the textbook does not deal adequately with a topic, additional readings might be necessary, e.g. when local figures and policies are not reflected in the textbook.
- When students are unlikely to experience a specific problem in their usual clinical placements, a field trip or classroom visit might be indicated. For instance, if there is a natural disaster in a rural area due to flooding, students might be assigned to do a field trip, since they are not likely to see a refugee situation in their usual community health placements.

In the light of the cost (both in time and money) of additional resources, a justification for their use is necessary.

Step 7: Choose an appropriate textbook

Textbooks are usually used to provide the students with a resource that covers the course content reasonably comprehensively. Although one would expect all tertiary level students to do additional readings, it is an economical use of their time to refer firstly to a standard textbook. Behar (1994) calls the textbook both the hub of the process of acquiring knowledge, and the link to other resources. She does point out that textbooks have important limitations, such as often leaving out controversies, and being too strongly focused on 'readability' rather than depth, and not acknowledging the ambiguity of knowledge.

It is important that teachers first develop their course, and then choose the textbook, and not use a textbook as a curriculum guide or lesson plan. Textbooks can contribute to curriculum choices, but should not be the curriculum.

It is a totally unsatisfactory situation to depend on extensive notes being taken down in class. The time of both the student and the teacher can be better utilized than for dictating notes.

When considering which textbook is the best for a specific course, the following may be considered:

- Is the content and approach in line with the objectives and framework of the course?
- Is the content accurate and based on current scientific evidence?
- Is the level of the textbook, both in terms of the depth and breadth of content covered and the language used, appropriate for the level of the course?
- Is the role of the nurse reflected in the textbook in line with the philosophy of the school?
- Do the print size, book size and illustrations contribute to understanding and usefulness?
- Is the textbook realistically priced in terms of the resources of the students?
- If no appropriate textbook is available, notes might have to be prepared for the course. In this case, the same criteria should be used to evaluate the notes. The course description should include a justification of the choice of textbook.

Step 8: Determine how students will demonstrate learning

Demonstration of learning in nursing is usually assessed by written tests and examinations, and by continuous clinical assessment and clinical examinations. Demonstration of learning should, however, be based on the expected learning outcomes, and the most appropriate format should be chosen to assess the specific outcomes. Asking a student to write how she/he will teach a client is not as valid an assessment method as actually seeing the student demonstrating this behaviour. The spirit and style of the assessment, as reflected through the demands of the various learning tasks, often is the best way of assessing whether superficial regurgitation type learning or deep understanding is the real aim.

Step 9: Write the course guide to be given to students

The format of the course guide is described below. It is an important document for both teacher and student, and as a first communication between the two parties, it should reflect the personality and philosophy of the teacher.

Step 10: Review

Before implementing the course, it should be reviewed by the Curriculum Committee, to ensure that it fits in with the overall curriculum, and by other colleagues for content validity. It is always useful to provide such reviewers with a written guide or questionnaire, so that you get systematic written feedback.

Step 11: Organize the course resources

This is the last step, and it involves everything from making sure that the textbooks are available, duplicating the course guide, booking the teaching venue, arranging classroom visits from experts, ordering additional references or audio-visual material for the library, and liaising with clinical settings. All these preparations are essential to make the course run smoothly.

The following components are useful in a course guide:

- *Course description:* This is a brief description of the course, which distinguishes it from other courses. It should correspond with the description given in the macro-curriculum and in the academic calendar of the educational institution.
- *Learning outcomes:* Course learning outcomes are more specific than level outcomes, and should relate to both the curriculum strands and the level and/or programme outcomes. Remember that the student should be able to use these specific learning outcomes to understand what breadth and depth of knowledge and what level of skill is required.
- *Course particulars:* This is the 'demographics' of the course, and includes the code, credit value, duration, prerequisites and periods scheduled for class and venue.
- *Learning/teaching methods:* A brief description is given of what learning experiences the student can expect, both inside and outside the classroom.
- *Expectations of students:* This section outlines for students what is expected of them. It includes both general expectations, for instance the level of class attendance and participation required, and specific expectation, for instance the assignments, the submission dates and the assessment criteria of each task.
- *Evaluation:* The components of the assessment should be listed, and the weighting of each towards the final evaluation given.
- *Schedule:* In this section a rough guide to the topics or units to be covered is given, sometimes with more specific unit learning outcomes and lists of resources applicable to the unit.
- *Contact details:* The teacher should give his/her name and title, as well as contact details. If the teacher is only available for consultation on specific days, this should be stated, and the procedure for making appointments outlined.

Unit planning

It is not usual for teachers at tertiary education institutions to have written teaching plans for every unit they teach. If one is working from a comprehensive course plan, in which the units are clearly delineated and the time planning (weighting) indicated, very little additional unit planning is necessary. For new teachers a more explicit unit plan may be useful.

A unit plan consists of the following:

Specific learning outcomes

These are based on the course learning outcomes, but are more specific. Usually a unit refers to a single course learning outcome, but it might also refer to more than one course learning outcome.

Task description

Describe how the student will use this part of the course in practice. Where does it fit in? What would be expected of the student?

Content

Identify which concepts, principles, skills and attitudes should be addressed in this unit.

Prerequisites

Identify what the student should bring into this unit, so that you can check this knowledge before commencing with the unit.

Presentation

The introduction of the classroom session: this may be a creative way of introducing a new topic, or it may review the previous work, to relate it to the new work.

Teaching methods

Decide how to approach the content, how much time to spend on each part of the unit, and how each part should follow the other. Also prepare teaching tools, such as videos, overhead transparencies, etc.

Evaluation

Prepare some times for tests and examinations based on this unit. Also prepare some discussion questions or criteria to evaluate classroom activities.

References

Make a list of the references used to prepare the unit. This might be useful if the content is challenged.

Course evaluation

Although curriculum review and evaluation are dealt with elsewhere, course evaluation will be dealt with here, for a number of reasons.

- **Course evaluation** Course evaluation is usually done every time a course is taught, and therefore done sooner in the course of a curriculum than the evaluation of the total curriculum.
- **The development** The development of the course evaluation mechanism and the management of the feedback received is often left to the individual teacher.
- **Designing the course** Designing the course evaluation mechanism while developing the course could help the teacher identify potential problems early.

A course evaluation is a systematic assessment of some or all aspects of the course in order to improve the course for future groups. If the teacher has implemented a specific innovation, or has become aware of a problem within the course, it might be appropriate to target the evaluation to the specific aspect of the course. If the course has been implemented for the first time, or if it is a known course without known problems, a more comprehensive evaluation might be indicated. If the teacher is doing the evaluation to support an application for promotion, or to add to her/his teaching portfolio, the evaluation might target the teacher's input specifically.

There are a number of agents who can be used for evaluation. Each has its own limitations and strengths.

- The teacher can do a self-evaluation, using existing evaluation instruments. This corresponds to the 'internal' evaluation of the curriculum, which is often a first step in curriculum evaluation. Take the instrument you are going to ask the external reviewers to use, and evaluate your own course. You may even prepare a report based on this evaluation, or make some changes based on this evaluation before going for external review.

- Past and present students can be asked to evaluate the course, based on a specific evaluation instrument. In a sense this can still be seen as 'internal' evaluation, since students are actually participants in the course. Students are the only people who can really directly evaluate the course as they have experienced it. They have usually had experience of many teachers, and therefore can compare and contrast, in order to evaluate the effectiveness of the course. The quality of evaluation from students can be improved by making sure one does not access a biased sample, and by also asking students some time after they have taken the course, so that they can evaluate the long-term usefulness of the course. It might be a good idea to allow current students to hand in the evaluation without identifying themselves, as this might lead to more honest feedback.
- Colleagues, such as level coordinators, or programme directors, can be asked to evaluate the course. This evaluation can be very useful, especially if you respect and like the colleagues, since this makes it easier to accept negative feedback.
- Empirical data can be used to evaluate the course. One can use existing data, such as measurement of student performance, or implement small evaluation projects and collect the required data. For instance, if you have changed the course to improve the writing ability of students, the results can be evaluated by comparing the writing skills of a previous group with the current group. This is more appropriate for targeted evaluation than for general evaluation.

The evaluation tools depend on the specific objectives of the evaluation. In general, the more junior the student, the more closed the items should be. Senior students and professional evaluators and colleagues usually appreciate more open-ended items, so that they can elaborate their opinions. In Figure 5.1, an example of a course evaluation of a nursing research course is given. The first element uses a rating scale to assess the student's satisfaction with different aspects of the course. The second item uses a semantic differential to assess the general attitude of the student towards the course. The last item asks the student to assess his/her competence in terms of the skills inherent in the course. Each item also allows for general comments with an open-ended item.

Clinical experience

The model of nursing education in the country, as described in Chapter 2, will have an enormous influence on the choice of clinical learning sites and experiences. If nursing is part of secondary education, the Curriculum Committee is constrained by the requirements of other subjects within secondary education. Similarly, if the school is a hospital school, the service needs might play a big role in the choices made.

Figure 5.1

An example: Course evaluation of a nursing research course

1. PLEASE RATE EACH OF THE FOLLOWING ASPECTS OF THIS COURSE BY MARKING THE APPROPRIATE BOX

	Very unsatisfactory	Unsatisfactory	Satisfactory	Very satisfactory
1. Course outline				
2. Essential readings				
3. Organization				
4. Content				
5. Teaching methods				
6. Teacher's attitude				
7. Teacher's knowledge				

Any other comments:

_____

_____

2. GIVE YOUR OPINION OF THE COURSE by making a cross anywhere on each line:

Stimulating	*———*———*———*———*	Boring
Very easy	*———*———*———*———*	Very difficult
Useful	*———*———*———*———*	A waste of time
Empowering	*———*———*———*———*	Disempowering
Confusing	*———*———*———*———*	Enlightening

3. PLEASE RATE YOUR COMPETENCE IN EACH OF THE FOLLOWING TOPICS

	I am sure I can do this	I think I understand	I don't think I understand	I am sure I don't understand
Formulating a problem, aims and objectives				
Finding relevant literature				
Doing a literature review				
Developing a conceptual framework or finding a theory for a study				

	I am sure I can do this	I think I understand	I don't think I understand	I am sure I don't understand
Identifying the appropriate research method				
Choosing an appropriate sample				
Developing an instrument				
Commenting on the validity and reliability of an instrument				
Calculating and interpreting average, standard deviation and reliability				
Developing tables				
Writing a proposal				
Making sure my research is ethical				
Writing a research article				

Any other comments:

_____

_____

The word 'clinical' actually refers to the bedside of the patient, but in the curriculum context it should be seen as learning the professional role and competence by doing practising under supervision in any healthcare setting. This means that in community health nursing, where the population, or a community, are the focus of nursing, the 'clinical' setting is not a hospital or a clinic, but could be a home, or a school, or a factory. The theoretical underpinnings of this component of the curriculum come from the experiential learning theory. This means that learning takes place in the real situation, with students as active participants and not just observers.

Clinical learning experiences are important for the following reasons:

1. It gives the student the opportunity for role learning as opposed to learning portions of the role, or pieces of theory. It is in clinical settings that the student learns what it means to be a nurse, or a community health nurse, or an intensive care nurse. Clinical experience is therefore also the only place where the student can learn contingency management competence, task management competence and role environment competence (see Chapter 4). These competencies, which form an integral part of role competence, cannot be taught or evaluated in a classroom setting. Some authors refer to

these three competencies as the contextualization of learning (Regehr and Norman, 1996).

2. Clinical experience gives the student the opportunity to apply learned knowledge and skills to the real situation. Without the opportunity to complete the learning cycle, as described by Kolb (1984), learning is not complete.

3. Although clinical experience depends to a large extent on previous class-room learning, there is an increasing understanding that much learning also takes place directly in the clinical setting. This refers particularly to role learning (point 1), but also to learning of new information and skills which form part of the technical competence of the role.

4. If one sees experiential learning in nursing as a form of service learning, the major benefit of that form of learning also applies to clinical learning in nursing. Service learning is defined as 'an educational activity that seeks to promote learning through experiences associated with community service (Howe, cited in Schine, 1997). Research shows that this form of learning promotes the social, psychological and intellectual development of students. They have a heightened sense of personal and social responsibility, enhanced self-esteem and moral growth.

5. Becoming competent depends on repeated practice of skills in a variety of situations. According to Benner (1984), a beginning practitioner needs to spend time in the practice setting to move from novice to competent practitioner.

While the major structuring of the clinical learning experiences will have been done by the Curriculum Committee, as part of the development of the macro-curriculum, the teachers developing the course should choose the specific health services to be used, and plan for the way they will be used.

Evaluating and choosing settings

In schools not directly affiliated with a particular hospital or service, educators have to choose appropriate clinical settings for the clinical learning experiences of their students.

In order to evaluate a service, one needs to do a site visit, and a situation analysis of the service. The following data should be collected about each service considered for inclusion in the programme:

- *Service rendered:* This should include an overview of general and special-ist services, and an evaluation of particular centres of excellence in the service.
- *Service utilization:* One needs to see to what extent the service is used by clients, since an under-utilized service might not provide adequate learning experiences for students.

- *Staff resources:* The assessment of staff resources should focus firstly on the staff who can function as role models for the students. If the programme aims to train clinical nurse specialists, it is ideal to find a service in which such nursing practitioners are already working successfully. Secondly, it should evaluate the general staffing levels, since these might influence student learning. For instance, if there is a severe shortage of surgeons, the surgical component of the pre-registration nursing programme might suffer.
- *Quality indicators:* Any situation analysis should include any data that can be found to indicate what the level of service in the institution is. If internal or external institutional quality review data are available, it should be accessed and used.
- *Other involvement in education:* Even the best service can be a poor learning experience if there are too many students placed there. This does not refer only to nursing or midwifery students, since students from other health professions often compete with nurses and midwives for learning opportunities. A comprehensive understanding of current student placements is therefore essential.

An example of a situation analysis form for the planning of a psychiatric nursing programme is available in Figure 5.2.

When choosing clinical settings for student placement, the following should be taken into account:

- *The level of support needed:* Not all settings provide equal support and supervision for students, or make equal demands on them. If junior students need a safe setting to practise, it is important to choose a setting where staffing is adequate, and which is close enough to the education institution to allow for frequent contact between students and teachers. If senior students need to develop self-confidence and independent decision-making, however, they might need a setting with fewer human resources and less support.
- *The specific competencies the course demands:* The course objectives are the guide used to identify what competence students should have the opportunity to practise. One should not choose clinical settings which do not allow these competencies to be practised by the students. Course developers should be careful not to make assumptions about what students will be able to do in certain settings. Their planned learning experiences have to be validated with the management of the service, and the practitioners in the unit. For instance, a number of new psychiatric patients might be seen in a psychiatric outpatient clinic every day. But if there is a policy that only registrars/psychiatry, do first interviews, psychiatric nursing students will not learn this competence in this setting. They might get more practice in this skill in a primary health care setting, where there are no registrars.

Figure 5.2

Situation analysis for psychiatric nursing course

Name of institution _____

Address _____

_____

_____

Postal code _____

Telephone number – area code _____ – _____

Fax number   – area code _____ – _____

Nurse in charge _____

1. PLEASE GIVE A SUMMARY OF THE PSYCHIATRIC SERVICES YOUR INSTITUTION PROVIDES:

1.1. OUTPATIENT CARE

Average nr of visits per month: _____

Are these numbers increasing? Yes_____ No_____ Not sure_____

If yes, please explain the extent and the possible reasons:

_____

_____

_____

Nr. of Psychiatric Nurses: _____ Nr. of Doctors: _____

Nr. of Psychiatrists: _____ Nr. of Psychologists: _____

Nr. of Social Workers: _____ Nr. of Occupational Therapists: _____

1.2 ADMISSION OR ACUTE CARE UNIT(s)

Nr. of beds in unit: _____ Nr. of units:_____

Average nr. of admissions per month: _____

Average nr. of discharges per month:_____

Most common diagnoses: _____

Nr. of Psychiatric Nurses: _____ Nr. of Doctors: _____

Nr. of Psychiatrists: _____ Nr. of Psychologists: _____

Nr of Social Workers: _____ Nr. of Occupational Therapists: _____

1.3 LONG-TERM OR REHABILITATION UNIT(s)

Nr. of beds in unit: _____ Nr. of units:_____

Average nr. of admissions per month: _____

Average nr. of discharges per month:_____

Most common diagnoses: _____

Main mode(s) of treatment: _____

Nr. of Psychiatric Nurses: _____ Nr. of Doctors: _____

Nr. of Psychiatrists: _____ Nr. of Psychologists: _____

Nr. of Social Workers: _____ Nr. of Occupational Therapists: _____

1.4 FORENSIC PSYCHIATRIC UNIT(s)

Nr. of beds in unit: _____ Nr. of units:_____

Average nr. of admissions per month: _____

Average nr. of discharges per month:_____

Most common diagnoses: _____

Main mode(s) of treatment: _____

Nr. of Psychiatric Nurses: _____ Nr. of Doctors: _____

Nr. of Psychiatrists: _____ Nr. of Psychologists: _____

Nr. of Social Workers: _____ Nr. of Occupational Therapists: _____

1.5 OTHER SPECIALIST AREAS:

Please list other specialist units in the hospital: _____

Nr. of beds in unit: _____ Nr. of units:_____

Average nr. of admissions per month: _____

Average nr. of discharges per month:_____

Most common diagnoses: _____

Main mode(s) of treatment: _____

1.6 COMMUNITY SERVICES

Which of the following community services are available for people living with a mental illness in your town/area?

Service	Yes	No
1. Primary health clinics offering outpatient care		
2. Support group for patients		
3. Support group for families		
4. Half-way houses or other residential services		
5. Special schools for children with mental retardation		
6. Counselling centre for children		
7. Counselling centre for adults		
8. Vocational rehabilitation centre		

2. PLEASE GIVE AN INDICATION OF TRAINING DONE IN YOUR INSTITUTION:

2.1 The number of students using the psychiatric units for training

Nursing students: _____ Medical students: _____

2.2 What other learning support or facilities would be available for students in your setting?

_____

_____

_____

2.3 Do you think your institution can provide adequate learning opportunities for psychiatric nursing training?

Yes: _____ No: _____

If not, what is inadequate? _____

3. OTHER

Is there anything else you would like to add?

_____

_____

_____

_____

_____

THANK YOU VERY MUCH FOR YOUR ASSISTANCE.

- *Central vs peripheral competencies:* Every course will cover such a large range of competencies that no single clinical setting will usually allow all of these to be practised. This limitation might be dealt with by rotating students through different settings, but rotating has to be done cautiously. If students remain in clinical settings for too short a period, they never learn the total role, but only fragments of it. They might also focus on skills or procedures, rather than understanding the type of service, and its demands on the nurse. Clinical placements should therefore be long enough to allow competence to develop. The range of competencies needed might also be dealt with by prioritizing competencies based on their importance to the role functioning of the practitioner. Clinical experiences are then chosen to focus on centrally important competencies. For instance, two medical units might be under consideration; one (unit 1) has a slower turnover, and deals with patients with chronic medical conditions, while the other (unit 2) has a high turnover, is extremely busy, and deals with patients with a very wide variety of medical conditions. If students need to learn patient and family health education, unit 1 might be the most appropriate. If senior students have to learn unit management of a demanding unit, unit 2 might be more appropriate.
- *Positive vs negative experiences:* It is important to make sure that the clinical experience that students have during their training does not leave them with negative perceptions of a particular field of nursing. For instance, in a specific school, students doing mental health nursing were placed in a long-term psychiatric hospital, where only 10% of their time was spent working with acute patients. In contrast, they spent 90% of their medical-surgical

time in acute units. Students therefore associated all the problems with chronic or long-term care only with mental health nursing, leading to a very poor uptake of post-graduate studies in this field of nursing. When the school changed the mental health nursing placement to primary health care settings, where students worked with families and ambulant clients, the attitudes changed dramatically.

- *Logistics:* Distance between the clinical facility and the school, the availability of student residences at distant services, and the availability of learning resources, such as computers and libraries, should also be considered when choosing clinical settings.
- *Equity:* Students should have different but equal learning opportunities in clinical settings. It is often not possible for the learning to be the same, but if a setting has some weaknesses, it should also have some strengths.

Examples of innovative clinical settings

Kendle, J. and Campanale, R. (2001) A pediatric learning experience. Respite care for families with children with special needs. *Nurse Educator*, **26**(2): 95–98.
Each student had to spend 14 hours giving respite care to children with special needs, ranging in age from 18 months to 14 years. This gave them the opportunity to learn this aspect of paediatric nursing, and also the skills of developing a professional relationship with families.

Brendtro, M. J. and Leuning, C. (2000) Nurses in churches: a population-focused clinical option. *Journal of Nursing Education*, **39**(6): 285–288.
This article describes the placement of students with parish nurses in three courses of a pre-registration programme. The role of the parish nurse includes health education, counselling, liaison to community resources, coordinating and teaching volunteers and dealing with the faith/health interface.

Organizing clinical learning

Once the clinical facilities have been chosen, the team should make sure that the necessary agreements are in place. This can take the place of a simple memorandum of understanding, setting out the agreement of the health service to accept a specified number of students from a specified programme for clinical learning experience in a specified setting for a specified time. It often spells out what is expected from the health facility, and also stipulates that students have to comply with the rules of the setting while in the placement. It should also stipulate the number of years for which it is valid, and how much notice should be given on either side when the placement is no longer available or no longer necessary to the school. In some settings a formal signed contract is required. This step is essential, so that the school is sure that the placement will not be withdrawn without giving adequate notice to make other arrangements for the students.

The next step is to communicate the intentions of the placement clearly to the staff in the units, and to the students and clinical facilitators. This is sometimes done by developing a set of learning outcomes for the clinical placement, or a list of role tasks the student has to master during the placement. This statement of the intended learning assists all concerned to work together towards the outcomes.

It is recommended that the clinical learning outcomes be part of the course description, in order for the clinical learning to be part of a holistic package of learning, and not a separate entity. Nursing is a science and an art. In the classroom the science is learnt, but in the practice setting the art is perfected. Seeing these two parts of the whole as separate entities leads to the misconception that one can be 'a good nurse, but cannot pass the examinations' or 'an excellent nursing student, but not good with patients'. A good nurse is a person who can use a thorough understanding of the knowledge-base of the discipline of nursing to care for people in a competent manner. Half of the whole is not 'good', it is totally inadequate.

The structure of the clinical learning facilitation should be outlined in the course description. Students should know who their clinical preceptors are, and what they can expect from them. They should also know what level of involvement they can expect from the staff of the unit in which they are placed. This information clarifies expectations, and also indicates to students that support is on hand. It is always a good idea to make maximum use of the expertise of the clinical staff, but it should be understood that patient care is the first priority of the staff, and they cannot be the only resource for students.

Lastly, one should develop the evaluation instruments to be used to assess the clinical competence of the students. This step should include formative evaluation as well as summative evaluation.

Record keeping

Although most higher education institutions keep careful records of the academic performance of students (courses passed, and marks achieved), it is only in professional schools where details of clinical learning experiences also need to be kept. The future registration of students with regulatory bodies, inside or outside the country, often depends on the records kept by the school.

To develop a student record, it is useful to study a number of registration forms from different countries where the students might want to register. This gives the developers of the student record a better idea of the level of detail that needs to be kept. Usually the number of hours of clinical learning in different types of settings needs to be recorded. The school should use a record that is completed on a monthly basis, and then is summarized at the end of the programme.

Conclusion

Course development is a creative process in which teachers can make the most of their understanding of the students, their enthusiasm for what they are teaching, and their view of the context of the teaching. A good course outline can become part of the portfolio of the teacher, and can be used for assessment when the person applies for promotion.

This outline is not, however, a document that can be rolled over from one year to the other. It is always a work in progress. It should be flexible, to accommodate changes in the situation and it should be amended after each use, to incorporate the feedback from students, and the new developments in the field.

Points for discussion

In his chapter on independent learning in Tait's 1994 anthology on open learning, Wright states that every course should aim to:

- encourage students to take more responsibility for their own learning, i.e. to become more independent as learners
- enable students to bring their own experiences to courses and to use these as sources of learning
- make the learning relate to the students' own needs and
- encourage a problem-centred orientation to learning (p. 123).

Take any course you have taken or developed, and discuss the extent to which it adheres to Wright's criteria.

References

Behar, L. S. (1994) *The Knowledge Base of Curriculum. An Empirical Analysis.* Lanham: University Press of America.

Benner, P. (1984) *From Novice to Expert: Promoting Excellence and Power in Clinical Nursing Practice.* Mento Part, CA: Addison-Wesley.

Glatthorn, A. A. (2000) *The Principal as Curriculum Leader. Shaping What is Taught and Tested.* Thousand Oaks, CA: Corrvin Press. Inc.

Kolb, D. A. (1984) *Experiential Learning.* Englewood Cliffs, NJ: Prentice Hall.

Regehr, G. and Norman, G. (1996) Issues in cognitive psychology: Implications for professional education. *Academic Medicine*, 71: 988–1000.

Schine, J. (ed) (1997) *Service Learning*. Chicago, IL: The National Society for the Study of Education.

Wright, T. (1994) Putting independent learning in its place. In Tait, A. (ed) *Key Issues in Open Learning – A Reader*. London: Longman.

Recommended reading

Broom, B. L. (2001) Assessing the value of the follow-through family project for students and families. *Journal of Nursing Education*, 40(2): 79–85.

When the time spent on a specific learning experience was challenged, faculty did a thorough evaluation of the cost and benefit to both students and families involved. The results were enough to convince faculty to keep the learning experience in the curriculum.

Chan, D. S. K. (2002) Associations between student learning outcomes from their clinical placements and their perceptions of the social climate of the clinical learning environment. *International Journal of Nursing Studies*, 39: 517–524.

This is a research article, which used the Clinical Learning Environment Inventory (CLEI) with 108 second year nursing students to explore the relationships between expectations and reality, and between learning environment and outcomes.

Chapter 6

Implementing a new curriculum

Nomthandazo S Gwele

Introduction

Implementing a new curriculum is never easy. Literature abounds on problems in, and/or barriers to, effective implementation of new curricula in educational institutions. Teachers' resistance to change, lack of knowledge and skills to implement the proposed change at classroom level and failure to gain teacher ownership of the new curriculum are some of the most frequently mentioned reasons for failure to effect change at classroom level (Glatthorn, 1981, Hord, 1987, 1992; Gwele, 1994). Effective implementation of a new curriculum is a function of (a) facilitative and visionary leadership, (b) an organizational culture and climate conducive to change, (c) evolutionary planning and coordinating of resources, (d) participant training and development, (e) monitoring and checking progress and (f) continued assistance and support (Hord, 1992).

Facilitative and visionary leadership

Hord (1992) provides a chronological analysis of change models in education. In the beginning, empirical-rational strategies, which placed emphasis on 'perfecting' the product or its parts were used. Then power-coercive strategies were used, which focused on changing the individual through power and coercion. These were followed by normative re-educative strategies, which were based on the belief that self-renewal and development were essential for effective adoption. Now a new type of change models, focusing on systemic or transformative change with appreciation of the role of facilitative curriculum leaders is beginning to emerge.

Literature abounds in definitions of leadership that differentiate positional from functional leadership, and management from leadership (Gardner, 1990; Hord, 1992; Mendéz-Morse, 1992). For instance Gardner (1990: 1) describes leadership as 'the process of persuasion or example, by which an individual (or leadership team) induces a group to pursue objectives held by the leader or shared by the leader and his or her followers'. Managers, on the other hand, are seen as individuals who 'hold a directive post in an organization, presiding over resources by which the organization functions, allocating resources prudently, and making the best possible use of people' (Gardner, 1990: 3). Whilst acknowledging the ideal and desirability of conceptions of leadership as a functional process rather than positional, or vested authority (Gardner, 1990; Hord, 1992; Owens, 1998) there is growing evidence that of all the factors that are essential for effective curriculum implementation, none are as significant as the principal or head of school or department (Boyd, 1992). Effective and successful implementation cannot occur without a visionary and facilitative leader and manager or principal. To this effect, Owens (1998: 217) contends that 'it is false to argue that . . . principals should be leaders, not managers, because they need to be both'.

Developing and sharing a vision

A head of school must have a vision and be able to articulate that vision to the staff, students and all stakeholders, including health services and the community served by the school of nursing. A vision is defined as 'mental pictures of what the school or its parts (programs, processes, etc.) might look like in a changed and improved state . . . a preferred image of the future' (Hord, 1992: 6). A comprehensive and communicable vision for curriculum innovation involves a vision of how the school might be in the future, what the leader aspires for the school as well as the processes and strategies necessary to effect the vision (Manasse, 1986). Curriculum implementation, however, is not only about the leader's vision but also about how well that vision is shared by the teachers and all those whose professional and/or personal lives will be directly or indirectly affected by the envisaged curriculum change. Curriculum planners and/or those in charge of nursing schools often fail to recognize teachers, students and health service management, as critical variables in effective implementation.

Adams and Chen (1981: 267) argued that 'for any innovation to gain the right of passage, it is essential to recognise the "greater relevant power"'. These authors further argued that many innovations have 'foundered at the work-face through simple but subtle opposition of teachers, who at that point, because they exercise effective control over what is done, constitute a source of relevant power (Adams and Chen, 1981: 268). In nursing education, students and the health services also constitute sources of relevant power. Implementation of a new curriculum in nursing will fail if students are not involved in decisions to change and health services will simply refuse to accommodate students on their facilities, if the services have no understanding of what the school is trying to achieve.

No dream or vision can occur to all people at the same time. The important thing to consider is not 'who thought about it first', but how the other role players were involved in the decision to implement the new curriculum. The vision begins as a rudimentary idea of what might be. Crystallizing and formulating the vision into tangible goals, processes and strategies must involve teachers, students, and the health service management at the very least. If the new curriculum involves using the community extensively as a clinical learning setting, then the community itself is a crucial stakeholder in the new curriculum and must also be an equal participant in the deliberations leading to decisions regarding the choice of a reform model to be used in effecting curriculum change.

Hord (1992: 4) warns that the 'actual selection of reform model, or combination of models, is one of the most important decisions the leadership team will make as it moves forward with comprehensive school reform. ... [and needs] a well-planned and carefully thought out process'. The same can be said for selecting a curriculum approach or model for nursing education in a particular nursing education institution.

Sharing the vision involves more than telling the institution's constituents what it is; sharing includes engaging them in interpreting the 'dream' as well as making decisions regarding making it reality. Deliberations on the vision should include an analysis of its educational, administrative and financial implications for the student and the school of nursing. Health service authorities will want to know what the change entails for health human resource development. Students and parents might want to know the value of the new curriculum with regard to graduates' employment opportunities, both nationally and internationally.

Educational implications

The teachers and all the other stakeholders need a clear understanding and appreciation of the expected learning outcomes, the congruency of the envisaged curriculum approach with the institution's philosophy of nursing and nursing education. The world over, nurse educators are being asked to ensure the development of life-long learning skills, inquiring and critical minds, as well as compassionate and caring nurses with a keen awareness of the interrelatedness of world politics, economy and global health. Changing from a traditional curriculum to a new and transformative curriculum that places emphasis on these educational outcomes might need a lot of defending and research-based argument to convince traditionalists that this is a 'good' thing to do.

Administrative implications

Some of the decisions made by educational institutions will be based mainly on administrative reasons rather than educational reasons. Issues such as the impact of the new programme on clinical learning facilities and classroom space must be taken into consideration when making decisions about a curriculum approach. Articulation of the programme structure with the parent institution's academic structure might mean changes and modifications of the initial 'vision'.

Financial implications

Change costs money. Questions such as 'Which is the most cost effective approach that can be used to attain the envisaged goals?', 'Can the school afford it?', 'Who is going to pay for it?', are all important. For example, as is indicated in the following chapters, PBL tends to be costly, both in terms of human and material resources. A nursing school with limited resources might ask if the educational outcomes that underpin PBL cannot be achieved by means of a case-based learning curriculum or a mixed curriculum. Starting with CBL in the first 2 years of a 4-year nursing programme and introducing PBL only in the last 2 years might be more appropriate for the questions such as 'How long will it take us to develop a new curriculum?' or 'Will we be able to implement a new curriculum next year?' are often asked. Figure 6.1 gives some idea of the preparation that needs to be done, and when and for how long it should be done. The figure also give some idea of the intensity of these activities over time.

Engaging the services of an external change facilitator

One of the important decisions that a school will have to make is whether to engage an external change facilitator or not. Havelock (1971) introduced the concept of change linkers acting as communication interface agents or agencies between developers and users. The 1970s were marked by a growth of evidence on the significance of facilitator(s) in facilitating and implementing change in education (Hord, 1992). It is believed that, initially, an external and independent consultant

Activities	Preparation		Implementation	Stabilization	
	Two years before implementation	One year before implementation	Year of implementation	One year after implementation	Two years after implementation
Planning	****	*****	****	*	*
Policy development	**	****	****	*	*
Gathering support for the programme	**	*****	****	**	**
Monitoring and evaluating the programme	**	**	***	**	**
Staff preparation and support	***	*****	*****	***	**
Student and stakeholder preparation and support	*	****	*****	***	***

* – Low intensity   ** – Moderate to low levels of intensity   *** – Moderate level of intensity
**** – High levels of intensity   ***** – Extreme levels of intensity

Figure 6.1 Tasks and task intensity before, during and after implementing a new curriculum

as a change facilitator is invaluable for any institution embarking on implementation of a major curriculum reform. As an 'outsider', the external expert carries no pre-conceived ideas about the staff's views about the envisaged change. The staff, on the other hand, know that this person is not linked to any decisions regarding their futures in the institution and they therefore are more likely to trust and be open with him/her regarding their concerns and learning needs pertinent to the new curriculum. The external change facilitator, however, has to ensure that by the time he/she leaves, adequate and relevant capacity has been built for internal facilitation to continue, without jeopardizing or undoing the work that had been achieved during his/her presence. The role of an external change facilitator in facilitating and monitoring implementation of a new curriculum is to:

- ensure common understanding of the new curriculum through discussion and dialogue with and among the staff and students
- assist the staff in locating and selecting relevant reading materials to help them develop the knowledge and skills required for competent implementation.
- assist the staff in identifying and locating other relevant resources in the form of other schools of nursing that have implemented a similar programme with whom the teachers can share experiences related to programme implementation.
- develop staff capacity to prepare students for their 'changed' roles through training, in the new curriculum. Students, similar to teachers, are often products of traditional teaching/learning environments, which demanded no more from them than that they listened, took notes, and reproduced what the teacher said in the classroom when required to do so. They will need orientation, preferably through workshops and simulated practice, in preparation for their roles in an active learning environment. Entrusting the responsibility for student training and development to the teachers ensures that the teachers' credibility among students regarding their ability to implement the new curriculum is not threatened
- provide technical support by assisting the teachers to develop the repertoire of knowledge and skills deemed to be necessary for effective classroom and clinical teaching/learning in the context of the new curriculum
- act as a liaison person or link agent between the teachers at operational level and management, in communicating those issues and/or problems which the staff see as managerial and/or administrative constraints to effective implementation.

Developing an organizational culture conducive to change

Organizational culture 'refers to shared philosophies, ideologies, values, assumptions, beliefs, expectations, attitudes, and norms that knit a community [an organization] together' (Owens, 1998: 165–166). Implicitly or explicitly members of the organization are socialized into the culture of the organization, which is what Owens refers to as 'the way things are done here' (1998: 166). Traditional single discipline nursing education institutions, such as colleges of nursing, tend to operate in a similar manner to primary and/or high schools. The timetable is often tight and packed with teacher-directed learning activities; nurse educators are often required to work office rather than academic hours. A new curriculum that purports to value self-directed learning and experimentation by students and teachers would not work well in such tightly regimented environments. Implementing a new curriculum, therefore, might necessitate more than a paradigm shift on the part of teachers and students. Systemic and structural change through dismantling institutional traditions and customs might be the most appropriate strategy in facilitating innovation. The head of a nursing department in a traditional university, or the principal of a nursing college governed by a bureaucratic and traditional health service department, might find it very difficult to effect curriculum change. Credibility of the principal and/or head of department as a hardworking and visionary leader and manager is invaluable in convincing those in authority that the envisaged curriculum change is important for the institution, positive student learning outcomes, the school and health human resource development.

Leadership at institutional and departmental level should recognize and encourage change, even within traditional institutions. Recognizing and acknowledging those teachers who dare take the risk to depart from custom and tradition signals a message that creativity and change are valued attributes in the school or department.

Evolutionary planning and resource allocation

Without careful and strategic planning even the most ideal curriculum change will not survive long enough to warrant assessment of its worth. Louis and Miller (cited in Hord, 1992) recommend evolutionary planning (moving step by step as the process unfolds) to 'blueprint' planning (working according to a rigid timetable and plan), perhaps for the simple reason that change is a process not an event (Hall and Hord, 1987; Hord, 1992). Evolutionary planning accepts that not every eventuality can be anticipated and planned for and that in most cases the outcomes and/or consequences of the planned change will require rethinking on the part of the planners.

'Providing resources has always been seen as the leader's role in change' (Hord, 1992: 7). Unless the leader has the authority (a head of school or principal), it might be difficult for the leader to fulfil this role. Curriculum change is dependent on sanctioning from those whose job it is to ensure prudent allocation of resources.

The institution must anticipate and budget for additional costs that implementing a new curriculum will place on the institution. Questions such as 'Will the department need to employ additional staff?', 'Will additional library and clinical learning resources be required?', 'How will students get to communities?' need to be confronted early. Avenues for raising the additional funds need to be explored. Experience has shown that most academic institutions will support a programme that has demonstrated its worth. Implementing a new curriculum will sometimes need external funding during the initial years of implementation until the parent institution has seen the gains for the institution as a whole, and is therefore ready to take over the financing of the programme.

Nevertheless, planning and providing resources involves more than money. It also includes planning time needed to effect the changes, releasing staff for training, materials development and other activities related to implementing the new curriculum. To be in the forefront of implementing a new curriculum can be both overwhelming and exciting to teachers. Management must be careful not to add to this feeling by not re-allocating some of the responsibilities of the implementation team to other staff members. It might be necessary to cut down on some of the school activities in order to ensure adequate planning. For instance, when the School of Nursing at the University of Natal decided to change from a traditional curriculum to PBL, the Head of School had to convince the university authorities that thorough planning necessitated that the school did not have a first year intake in the year preceding implementation. Furthermore, the school had to forego a social science major as a second major in the pre-registration nursing degree. Such decisions had to be based on the shared vision of the school and its pre-registration education programme, which placed emphasis on the school establishing itself as an innovative and dynamic School of Nursing, recognized as a centre of excellence in nursing and midwifery education in Africa. Above all, effort must be placed on concentrating resources where they will make a difference in student learning (Boyd, 1992; Fullan, 1985; Hord, 1992).

Providing participant training and development

Staff development has been conceptualized as a 'tool for improving educational vitality of . . . institutions through attention to the competencies needed by individual teachers and to the institutional policies required to promote excellence' (Wilkerson and Irby, 1998: 390). No institution will decide on a 'carbon copy' of an educational programme in another institution. Educational programmes bearing similar names or titles, for example PBL or CBE, will differ according to the context in which they are offered. Each institution, however, will embark on staff development activities aimed at promoting excellence in teaching and learning in line with its philosophy, history, culture and economic status.

Irrespective of whatever implementation strategy is employed, 'ideally everybody all along the line ought to be fully competent at their respective jobs. Such an ideal state of affairs seldom exists, although there are some countries . . . that operate on the (optimistic) assumption that it does' (Adams and Chen, 1981: 253). It has been noted elsewhere that, although no amount of training and preparation can ever adequately prepare teachers for the unintended and unanticipated outcomes of implementing a new curriculum, the significance of the process of learning and re-socialization when implementing an innovation that demands a radical departure from custom and tradition cannot be over-emphasized. Failure to provide time and opportunity for nurse educators to acquire the new repertoire of skills and knowledge they need to implement the new curriculum may lead to inadequate implementation and rejection of the new curriculum (Dalton, 1988). A process of learning and re-socialization is essential in order to prevent feelings of inadequacy to meet the demands of a new curriculum. Nurse educators need a sustained and continuous effort to help them come to terms with what needs to be changed and how it should be changed (Gwele, 1994). Preparing staff for implementing a new curriculum is the most important single strategy for successful change and no nursing education institution can afford to neglect it. The cost of failure to provide staff with learning opportunities so that they are well equipped to assume their changed roles is enormous, both emotionally and financially.

The participant development process

Staff training efforts should take into consideration that staff are never at the same level of development regarding any innovation. Some staff are passionate readers and seekers of new knowledge and developments in the practice of nursing education, while others are 'routine'-oriented people and are happy going to the classroom, doing the same thing, the same way, year in and year out. A comprehensive staff development approach, taking into account the diverse development needs of staff is essential. Most programmes would need to cater for (a) entry level teachers; (b) advanced level teachers; (c) educational programme leaders; and (d) teacher scholars (Wilkerson and Irby, 1998). It stands to reason that those who have never taught before, irrespective of the new curriculum approach, will need a different kind of programme, at least in levels of intensity, compared to advanced teachers, who might require more focus on what they need to do differently from what they have been doing over the years. Similarly, programme directors or curriculum leaders need development activities focusing on managing and facilitating change, in addition to knowledge and skills related to teaching/learning strategies, whereas the scholar teachers might need some guidance in accessing available research and prevailing theoretical discourses on the new curriculum programme.

Obtaining base-line data on staff readiness to implement a new curriculum

Analysis of staff concerns about change before implementation helps provide base-line data against which the progression or development of concerns about the new curriculum can be measured.

Base-line data on staff readiness to implement the new curriculum help focus development activities on staff needs and concerns. The concerns-based adoption model (CBAM: Hall and Hord, 1987) and the framework on the levels of influence on the teaching/learning process (Trigwell, 1995) have proved to be very useful for obtaining such information on staff preparedness for facilitating implementation of a new curriculum. One of the foundational principles of the CBAM is that change 'is a highly personal experience' and that it is 'accomplished by individuals first, then by institutions' (Hord, 1992: 11).

Experience has shown, however, that unless data on teachers' conceptions about teaching, their planning for teaching, as well as their teaching activities are obtained, the tendency is to provide technical staff development programmes, which focus only on teaching strategies (Gwele, 2000; Trigwell, 1995). When the new curriculum requires a complete paradigm shift, examining teachers' conceptions about teaching affords teachers an opportunity to reflect on their values and beliefs about teaching and learning and examine those in the light of the proposed new curriculum and the philosophy of the school. According to Trigwell (1995) the institutional context, teachers' conceptions about teaching, learner characteristics and teacher characteristics, all act together to influence student learning. There is very little if anything at all, that one can do to address teacher and learner characteristics. Conceptions about teaching, however, present a challenge for staff development workers and change facilitators in education, because for teaching practice to change, conceptions about teaching need to change first. Table 6.1 provides an illustration of the relationship among conceptions about teaching, conceptions about learning, planning and teaching strategies.

Creating space for staff to reflect and deliberate on their conceptions of teaching and concerns about the new programme

Once the data on staff concerns, values and practices have been analysed, opportunities must be created for both individual and group feedback. During the individual feedback, focus should be on the individual and not the whole group. With the individual teacher, the change facilitator identifies areas that need focus and attention for development, as well as strategies for dealing with concerns. The teacher should be asked to identify what he/she will do to deal with identified concerns as well as what he/she expects the institution to do to help him/her deal with concerns regarding the new curriculum. Evidence has shown that when this is not done, teachers tend to expect the school to deal with 'their' concerns and not see themselves as also instrumental in the process of trying to resolve concerns (Gwele, 1997; 2000).

The change facilitator should be warm and responsive in working with teachers (Berk and Winsler cited in Sheerer, 1997). Change can be very threatening to individuals. Teachers take years learning their classroom skills and to be told that they have to learn new skills might be very unsettling; hence the need

Table 6.1 Conceptions about teaching and learning, and related planning and teaching strategies

Teaching as	Learning as	Planning for teaching	Teaching strategies
Transmission of information	Memorization and acquisition of information, e.g. signs and symptoms of disease.	An outline of important concepts and facts A handout with 'important' information	Lecturing
Facilitating the development of inquiring minds	An interpretive and inquiry process	Anecdotes of real-life experiences embedded in what needs to be learned An outline of important questions to be asked	Interactive strategies – discussion, role plays, questioning
Facilitating critical reflection through a dialogical process*	Meaning making through critical analysis and reflection on meaning perspectives about health and disease, nursing, caring, etc	Anecdotes of real life experiences embedded in what needs to be learned An outline of reflective and critical questions to be asked focusing on meaning Careful attention to seating arrangement (face-to-face)	Debates, discussions, field-based learning, seminars, etc.
Helping students learn how to learn*	An emancipatory and lifelong process	Anecdotes of real-life experiences embedded in what needs to be learned An outline of reflective and critical questions to be asked focusing on meaning Careful attention to seating arrangement (face-to-face)	Debates, discussions, field-based learning, seminars, etc.

*Although these two approaches use the same strategies, the outcomes may be different.

to take teachers' concerns seriously. Some may seem minor to the change facilitator, but these concerns will be real and important to those who raise them, otherwise there would be no need to mention them.

Group feedback helps the discussion to focus on those aspects that are common to all staff members. Frequently occurring concerns and conflicting views between the school's espoused philosophy of education and staff views about teaching, planning and strategies form the basis for staff development activities targeting the whole school rather than the individual.

Providing individualized and targeted staff training and development

Glatthorn (1981) and Wilkerson and Irby (1998) discuss some of the strategies which may be used for staff development. A number of faculty development programmes have placed emphasis on collaborative and interactive approaches to staff development (Tiberius, 1995). Of essence is that whatever strategy is selected it has to be congruent with the basic tenets of the new curriculum about teaching and learning. Classroom observation, peer coaching for teaching improvement and workshops seem to be the most commonly used strategies for staff development.

The value of individualized staff development in implementing a new curriculum is well documented (Sheerer, 1997). Based on Vygotsky's socio-cultural theory of learning, Sheerer (1997) demonstrates how the concept of zone of proximal development (ZPD) can be used to improve in-service education programmes. The ZPD refers to the difference between what the individual learner can do on his/her own and that which he/she can learn to do with the help of peers and/or the change facilitator, a process which Vygotsky refers to as 'scaffolding'.

The most direct method for the change facilitator to use in helping teachers to monitor and assess their own teaching practice is to watch them in action in a classroom. This classroom observation offers an opportunity to observe an individual teacher in action, identify his/her strengths and jointly design a programme of action. Agreement about classroom observations and use or non-use of video tapes for observation and discussion must be reached. It is important that classroom observations are not carried out by someone with supervisory responsibilities in the school. Being observed while teaching is unnerving under ordinary circumstances, and it could be worse when one is experimenting with something new. It should be made clear to teachers that classroom observation is solely for teaching improvement practices and not for performance appraisal. Classroom observation should be followed by discussion with the individual teacher. Teachers must be encouraged to analyse and comment on their own performance before the change facilitator comments. Teachers tend to focus on the negative aspect of their performance and attribute effective behaviours to students rather than their own actions in the classroom. The change facilitator should re-direct the teacher to talk about the positive aspects first, as well as identify those actions which might have contributed to positive student performance. The areas that need improvement are then identified jointly with the teacher and plans are made for helping the teacher attain his/her goals for teaching improvement. Table 6.2 presents a checklist that could be used for classroom observation aimed at teaching improvement rather than performance evaluation. The main feature of this checklist is that, as a formative assessment tool, it is not designed for grading performance but rather to observe and record performance.

Table 6.2 A checklist for classroom observation

A. QUESTIONING

Types of questions	*By the teacher*	*By the students*
Factual questions		
Clarification questions		
Cause and effect or linkage questions		
Comparative questions		
Evaluative questions		
Critical questions		
Process questions		

B. OTHER ASPECTS OF EFFECTIVE TEACHING PRACTICE

Focusing the session

Discernible sequence of events

Asks questions aimed at monitoring students' understanding of what is taught

Students allowed time to think

Redirects questions to other students

Students asked to evaluate their responses and/or contributions

Assigns work for independent learning in preparation for next class session

C. GROUP PROCESS

Most students participated in the class session (approximately 80%)

Deals with disruptive students

Deals with domineering students

Encourages non-participants to take part in class discussion

Holds students responsible for own learning (assesses learning from work done outside class)

General comments

Types of questions adapted from McKeachie (1994) and aspects of effective teaching practice adapted from Hopkins (1993).

It is essential that the teacher is kept at his/her zone of proximal development ZPD during the whole process of staff development. Individual assessment and monitoring helps the change facilitator and the teacher gain a clear understanding of what the teacher is able to do on his/her own as well as what he/she needs expert guidance on. Guidance should continue only as long as it is needed by the teacher, and the change facilitator should begin to let go as soon as the teacher demonstrates ability to work on his/her own. The aim is to promote self-regulation, and therefore, one of the essential skills for any change facilitator is to recognize when his/her services are no longer needed. The process of individual consultation and discussion between the change facilitator and the teachers should help the teachers learn how to monitor and assess their own practice, identify their own learning needs and decide on actions that need to be taken in order to deal with identified learning needs.

Peer coaching for teaching improvement refers to a collaborative arrangement between two colleagues who volunteer to observe each others teaching practice and provide each other with formative feedback (Wilkerson and Irby, 1998). Use of peers for classroom observation depends on extremely trusting and confidence-inducing environments. The teachers must be allowed freedom to choose to use this strategy. Peer coaching has not been successful where it has been viewed as an expectation or requirement rather than a choice that teachers could exercise from among many other options.

Targeted training applies to group learning as well. More often than not there will be those aspects of implementing a new curriculum which most or all of the teachers need more knowledge and skills in order to implement. Longer and continuous staff training and development programmes utilizing 3–5 day workshops spread over time seem to work better than shorter and 'one-shot' workshops (Glatthorn, 1981; Wilkerson and Irby, 1998).

Staggering the duration of workshops, based on what needs to be done, works effectively from the author's experience. A week-long workshop at the beginning, focusing on information, dialogue and persuasion for the first day or two, followed by refining of the implementation plan as well as skills development for the remainder of the week seems to work well. It is unlikely that everyone will have accepted the new curriculum at this stage. It is therefore one of the responsibilities of the change facilitator (preferably external to the school) to 'sell' the new programme, as well as provide as much information as possible, starting from the beginning, reinforcing the reasons for change, the school's vision for the organization, the future and the personal aspirations of the advocates of the new curriculum about the school. Subsequent workshops of 2–3 days, targeting identified staff learning and development needs should be carried out at 3–6 month intervals, to allow enough time for staff to monitor their progress as well as seek alternative avenues for assistance and thus ensure self-direction in learning and problem-solving. Staff should be made aware that, except for the initial workshop, all workshops will focus on skill development rather than information acquisition.

Some of the principles of Vygotsky's socio-cultural learning theory (joint problem-solving and intersubjectivity), although based mainly on children's learning, apply just as well to adult learning (Berk and Winsler cited in Sheerer, 1997).

- Joint problem-solving – nurse educators, through simulated practice, self critique and group critique, learn to solve problems related to the new skill together. Simulated practice and demonstration provide a non-threatening environment for nurse educators to try their newly learned knowledge and skills, with the help of constructive feedback from colleagues.
- Intersubjectivity – a process of trying to achieve common understanding of the innovation. For instance, a number of people hold different conceptions of PBL, and PBL has been applied differently at different schools. A group workshop helps clarify concepts and constructs embedded in the new curriculum, to ensure common understanding within the school and the programme.

Monitoring and checking progress

The role of the teacher scholars and the curriculum leaders, in facilitating and monitoring the process of implementing a new curriculum cannot be over-emphasized. The external facilitator must ensure partnership with this group of curriculum leaders in the school. In fact, these teachers should be part of the curriculum development committee, because without partnership and collaboration with them, the external change facilitator cannot succeed in his/her role. Working together with this group of teachers, the change facilitator must ensure that implementation data are collected, analysed, interpreted and fed back to the school as a whole. Continuous sharing and discussion of the implementation data with the whole staff helps maintain the feeling of ownership by the entire school. Failure to communicate information to the whole staff might lead to lack of support for the new programme from those teachers who are not part of the teaching team. An 'us' and 'them' situation is not conducive to effective change.

Management also has to be part of the process. Some of the problems identified during implementation might need intervention by management. If management is not part of the process it might be impossible to make the changes necessary for effective implementation, especially if such changes involve systemic or structural changes, re-allocation of resources and/or changes in staff work assignments.

Monitoring and process evaluation should be built into the implementation plan. Decisions regarding what data will be collected, to what purpose, how and when, must be made before the programme is implemented. Fullan (1985) recommends that data on the state of classroom practice or implementation, factors affecting implementation, and outcomes with regard to student learning, skills and attitudes of the teachers constitute some of the essential data that need to be collected in monitoring implementation. In nursing education, essential implementation monitoring will also include data on attitudes and skills of clinical staff responsible for facilitating student learning in clinical learning sites, as well as the views of the students regarding the new programme and its implementation. The value of monitoring the implementation process lies in the fact that it ensures that problems are identified and dealt with timeously. Also, it conveys a message to the implementers that the school cares about what they are doing and wants to help them succeed.

Continued assistance and support

Often curriculum innovations fail after the initial three to four years of implementation due to lack of continued support and assistance. Most probably, the external change facilitator will have long left the institution by this time. It is the duty of the curriculum leaders to take over where the external agent left off. Staff turnover, lack of stimulation from new developments and ideas are just some of the reasons why most innovations lose their 'novel' status, and staff find themselves lapsing into that which was familiar and routine. As the staff gain the basic knowledge and skills required to achieve competence in implementing the new curriculum, they will need room to experiment and test new ideas founded on their experiences with the new curriculum. They need to feel that it is safe to do so and that assistance is available to them to discuss and test their ideas. A truly transformative curriculum does not expect uniform implementation from teachers, but rather that in time the uniqueness of each teacher as a practitioner will be evidenced in his/her teaching practice, without negating the school's philosophy of education and the programmes' expected learning outcomes.

Conclusion

There are no 'blueprints' for effective implementation of a new curriculum. Often the organizational context, staff expertise and the healthcare delivery system will determine the process of implementation in a particular institution. A number of factors, however, remain constant, in whatever situation one finds oneself. A facilitative visionary leader who knows how to balance pressure and support, an environment that openly values change and creativity, staff training and development as well as continued monitoring and support will go a long way towards creating and improving conditions for effective implementation of a new curriculum.

Points for discussion

1. If you are a nurse educator, but not heading a School or Department, and you are interested in changing the curriculum, how could you go about initiating curriculum change?
2. f you are involved in a process of curriculum change, which aspects of your new curriculum:
    *   have been thoroughly evaluated and described in the literature?
    *   have not been properly evaluated and described?
    How can you build such evaluation into your implementation process?

References

Adams, R. S. and Chen, D. (1981) *The Process of Educational Innovation: An International Perspective*. London: Kegan Page.

Boyd, V. (1992) *School Context: Bridge or Barrier to Change*. Southwest Educational Development Laboratory. Online. Available at: http://www.sedl.org/change/school/ (accessed 1 April 2004).

Dalton, T. H. (1988) *The Challenge of Curriculum Innovation: A Study of Ideology and Practice*. Philadelphia: Farmer Press.

Fullan, M. G. (1985) Change processes and strategies at the local level. *The Elementary School Journal*, 85: 391–422.

Gardner, J. W. (1990) *On Leadership*. New York: The Free Press.

Glatthorn, A. A. (1981) Curriculum change in loosely coupled systems. *Educational Leadership*, 38: 110–113.

Gwele, N. S. (1994) *The Process of Change in Nursing Education in South Africa*. A PhD thesis, Durban, South Africa: University of Natal.

Gwele, N. S. (1997) The development of staff concerns during implementation of problem-based learning in a nursing program. *Medical Teacher*, 19: 275–284.

Gwele, N. S. (2000) Facilitating and monitoring implementation of a case-based curriculum. In K. Appleton, C. Macpherson, and D. Orr (eds) *Selected Papers: Lifelong Learning Conference*, Yeppoon, Queensland, Australia. Hosted by Central Queensland University, July 2000.

Hall, G. E. and Hord, S. M. (1987) *Change in School: Facilitating the Process*. Albany, NY: State University of New York Press.

Havelock, R. G. (1971) *Planning for Innovation through Dissemination and Utilization of Knowledge*. Ann Arbor, MI: University of Michigan, Institute for Social Research.

Hopkins, D. (1993) *A Teacher's Guide to Classroom Research*. Buckingham, UK: Open University Press.

Hord, S. M. (1987) *Evaluating Educational Innovation*. London: Croom Helm.

Hord, S. M. (1992) *Facilitative Leadership: The Imperative for Change*, Southwest Educational Development Laboratory. Online. Available at: www.sedl.org/change/ facilitate/ (accessed 1 April 2004).

Manasse, A. L. (1986) Vision and leadership: paying attention to intention. *Peabody Journal of Education*, 63(1): 150–173.

McKeachie, W. J. (1994) *Teaching Tips: Strategies, Research, and Theory for College and University Teachers*. Toronto, Canada: D.C. Heath and Company

Mendéz-Morse, S. (1992) *Leadership Characteristics that Facilitate School Change.* Southwest Educational Development Laboratory. Online. Available at: http://www.sedl.org/change/leadership/ (accessed 1 April 2004).

Owens, R. G. (1998) *Organizational Behavior in Education.* Boston, MA: Allyn and Bacon.

Sheerer, M. (1997) Using individualization and scaffolding to improve inservice programs. *Early Childhood Education Journal*, 24: 201–203.

Tiberius, R. G. (1995) From shaping performances to dynamic interaction: the quiet revolution in teaching improvement programs. In: W.A. Wright et al. (eds) *Teaching Improvement Practices: Successful Strategies for Higher Education.* Bolton, MA: Anker Publishing Company.

Trigwell, K. (1995) 'Increasing faculty understanding of teaching. In: W.A. Wright et al. (eds) *Teaching Improvement Practices: Successful Strategies for Higher Education.* Bolton, MA: Anker Publishing Company.

Wilkerson, L. and Irby, D. (1998) Strategies for improving teaching practices: a comprehensive approach to faculty development. *Academic Medicine*, 73(4): 387–395.

Recommended reading

Gwele, N. S. (1997) The development of staff concerns during implementation of problem-based learning in a nursing program. *Medical Teacher*, 19: 275–284.

This article describes a study using the concern-based adoption model to track staff concerns during implementation of a new curriculum.

Mawn, B. (2000) Reconfiguring a curriculum for the new millennium: the process of change. *Journal of Nursing Education*, 39(3): 101–108.

This article describes the process of changing a curriculum in a university school of nursing.

Chapter 7

Curriculum evaluation

Marilyn B Lee

Introduction

Programme evaluation is often done as an after-thought to planning and implementing a new curriculum. This is unfortunate, since early planning of the evaluation allows for appropriate data collection early in the process. Programme evaluation is also sometimes the result of challenges from inside or outside the school about the quality of the programme, or it might be a requirement from the regulatory body or higher education authorities.

In this chapter the definitions, purpose, types and steps in evaluation are followed by an introduction to several common curriculum evaluation models.

Curriculum evaluation

Curriculum evaluation is usually a systematic, summative examination of all components of a curriculum that results in evaluative conclusions, such as approval or accreditation. The findings are used to develop, maintain and/or revise the programme (Loriz and Foster, 2001; UNFPA, 2001). In many instances social science research methods are used.

Evaluation is designed to assess the logic and coherence of curriculum concepts, design, implementation and utility (Herbener and Watson, 1992). Some evaluation models focus on judgement while others are more developmental in their orientation.

A number of principles should underpin any programme review: 'fairness, objectivity, comprehensiveness, credibility, usefulness and effective communication' (Thomas et al., 2000). These principles are needed to ensure that the review is authoritative and is given the consideration it deserves.

Collaboration in development of the standards and criteria as a first step in the review process ensures that contextual characteristics, such as culture, are taken into consideration when reviewing a programme. Furthermore, collaboration fosters trust and respect and reduces the threat that often results from review and evaluation (Lusky and Hayes, 2001; Thomas et al., 2000). Finally, collaboration may enhance the validity of data obtained through an evaluation (Hopkin, 2003).

The purpose of curriculum evaluation

In general, the purpose of an evaluation is to see if the programme or curriculum is doing what it is supposed to do or to determine the quality of the programme. The concept of quality as fitness for purpose is common, and determination of level of quality is a major reason for programme evaluation (Gilroy et al, 2001; Thomas et al., 2000).

In any curriculum evaluation there are usually specific questions that the evaluator or reviewer wishes to answer by performing the evaluation. Examples are: How well prepared graduates are to take employment in health care institutions? or What teaching strategies are being used to ensure that the graduate is prepared to make sound clinical judgments? The answers to these questions are typically used to make decisions about modifications in policy or programme (UNFPA, 2001).

Specific questions used in evaluation usually focus on one or more of the following issues: (a) accountability; (b) improvement; and (c) programme marketing (Priest, 2001). These issues are further described below.

Accountability

The most fundamental reason for evaluation and review of nursing programmes is protection of the public or accountability to stakeholders. Stakeholders are those individuals, groups or organizations that have an interest in something (UNFPA, 2001). In this case, stakeholders include students (who are, in fact, products of the programme), staff in the educational institution, staff in the healthcare facilities that employ the graduates, and government or non-governmental agencies that employ graduates from the programme or that make decisions relating to nursing education and practice.

Quality of nursing care is expected to be, at least partially, a result of the quality of the education of nurses (Crotty, 1993). Therefore, most stakeholders consider educational programmes accountable for the quality of nurses produced. Good quality programmes are more likely to result in good quality nursing care in a community. Moreover, protection of the public through good quality nursing care is one of the most essential purposes of professional regulatory bodies and therefore review and evaluation of nursing programmes often rests with or is delegated to these bodies. This is the case in many countries in North America (Canada and the USA), Australia, Europe and Africa. In contrast, some countries have non-professional bodies that perform the role of review and/or evaluation of health educational institutions or programmes, i.e., university senates or councils. Regardless of who performs the evaluation it is clear that evaluation is essential to ensure quality of programmes and the graduates that are produced.

Improvement

A second issue addressed by evaluation is improvement. A systematic evaluation can provide programme leaders with evidence of the strengths and weaknesses in a programme for improved teaching and learning practices, value of the experience, and professional competency. In addition, evaluation can support testing of innovations, reduce stakeholder concerns and establish programme standards or benchmarks (Priest, 2001). This 'improvement-focused' model (Prosavac and Carey, 1997) of programme evaluation is useful in improving the effectiveness of evaluation in continuous quality improvement.

Marketing

The third major issue that evaluation is concerned with is the marketability of a programme and its graduates. Until recently, higher education was protected from the global competitive market. This is especially true of public higher education institutions, as the massification of higher education ensured that the supply of students was continuous. What has changed, however, is the decrease in public funds for higher education and the concomitant increase in learners who look for the greatest value for their money. The increase in asynchronous delivery methods (virtual or distance universities) ensures that learners can continue to work while earning higher education qualifications. More and more institutions of higher learning are finding that there is a need for marketing their programmes, which includes evaluation of programmes and the dissemination of results of evaluations to ensure quality to stakeholders.

Types of evaluation

There are a number of characteristics of curriculum evaluation. Those that are included in this discussion are listed below with a discussion of each of the characteristics.

- internal versus external
- formative versus summative
- holistic versus specific
- high stakes versus low stakes
- degree of participation by stakeholders.

Internal versus external

Review and evaluation can be either internal or external. Internal means that the process of evaluation occurs within the institution and is usually a reflective process. External review or evaluation is performed by an outside agency, often using specific predetermined measures of quality (standards or benchmarks).

Many programmes have mechanisms in place to ensure that both internal and external review and evaluation take place. For example, there may be a continuous internal process of curriculum review with a periodic external process for evaluation of a curriculum. Systems such as this, which exists at the University of Botswana, usually are formal in nature and have senate-approved mechanisms for assessment, including specific components of a curriculum to be assessed. Standards and criteria for measuring performance, however, may be set centrally (by senate) or departmentally (at the programme level). In the case of the University of Botswana, minimum standards are set and the departments which offer the programmes identify continuous improvement criteria.

Standards and criteria used in external review may be specific with regard to expectations in specific curriculum areas such as programme delivery or student assessment, while other external evaluations may be conducted to determine that quality control and assurance mechanisms are in place within a programme. For example, a reviewer may want to be assured that mechanisms are in place to guarantee that student assessment is fair and valid, i.e., processes of internal or external moderation of assessments after development (setting) and after students have completed the assessment (marking). In the African region of the World Health Organization a set of standards for nursing and midwifery education has been developed and tested by the regional office. The Africa Honour Society for Nursing has also set up a process of internal and external review, which is available to schools in the region. In many individual countries, external reviews are done by the regulatory body for nursing and midwifery, or by the state department under which they are run (e.g., Department of Education, or Department of Health).

Formative versus summative

As previously mentioned, review and evaluation can be formative or summative. In general, review processes are formative in that they allow discovery of strengths and weaknesses for the purpose of continuous quality improvement, while evaluations are summative for the purpose of judgement, i.e., approval or accreditation by a professional body. An example of summative evaluation is the nursing council accreditation or approval visits. Summative evaluations are periodic and are usually done on 5–7 year cycles (Perry, 2001).

Holistic versus specific

Reviews and evaluations can be holistic or specific. An holistic evaluation is one in which all elements of the curriculum are considered. Reviews that are specific to a particular aspect of the curriculum are often referred to as audits. For example, a curriculum may be reviewed to see if the regulations are being implemented as described in the programme documents. Audits, especially internal audits, are generally done for two purposes: (a) identification or description of a problem and (b) recommendation of solutions.

Degree of participation

In any review or evaluation there may be varying degrees of participation by stakeholders, i.e., participation may occur at specific stages of the evaluation and/or different stakeholders may participate at different times. The level of participation by stakeholders may vary from low to high. It is best if decisions about participation are made at the outset but in some cases this is not possible. There should, however, be flexibility in the process, to allow for varying degrees of participation. High participatory evaluation implies that the stakeholders help to determine what is to be evaluated, how it should be evaluated and how the findings should be used. Participatory evaluations are particularly useful in producing collective learning and capacity building (UNFPA, 2001). This type of evaluation is also very useful where external review teams are responsible for evaluation, since the stakeholders generally have a better knowledge of the peculiarities or contextual factors that impact on a curriculum.

What to evaluate

It is generally agreed that a curriculum consists of: philosophy and/or mission, conceptual framework, goals, role description of the graduate, programme outcomes, level or year outcomes, course descriptions, content, and teaching and assessment strategies (Gerbic and Kranenburg, 2003). Other aspects that often are included in a curriculum are academic regulations of the department or institution, learning resources and plans for evaluation of the programme. There is, however, much variation in the agreed components of curriculum that should be included in evaluation and review. All stakeholders in and outside the organization should agree to the processes and content to be included in the curriculum review or evaluation. Furthermore, areas of review and evaluation used by the regulating body for nursing education in the country should be considered when determining what aspects of the programme to evaluate.

Evaluation of a new or revised educational programme is an integral part of curriculum planning and should be considered a part of development of the curriculum (Chevasse, 1994). Moreover, in evaluation of a curriculum, consideration must be given to all features of the curriculum, i.e., content, processes and outcomes. It is also suggested that an understanding of the issues related to implementation of the curriculum is essential and involves an in-depth, critical analysis of the problems, i.e., strengths and weakness in the system(s), and this analysis may include any part of the curriculum (Sutcliffe, 1992).

Planning for evaluation

The following questions need to be asked and answered in planning for evaluation (UNFPA, 2001):

- What is the purpose of the evaluation or review?
- What should be evaluated? Are there specific standards or benchmarks? For what purpose will the findings be used? What resources are needed?
- How do we evaluate this? What data are required and how can we collect them?
- Who will do the evaluation? Is outside consultation required? Who will use the data obtained?
- When will the evaluation be done? When should results and recommendations be expected?

These questions need to be thoroughly discussed and decisions taken, if the evaluation is to be useful.

Steps in an evaluation

An evaluation normally consists of the following steps.

- defining the standards
- investigating the performance or data collection
- synthesizing the results
- formulating recommendations
- feeding recommendations and lessons learned back into the programme.

The following section describes each of these steps in more detail.

Step one: defining the standards

Data obtained from review or evaluation are usually compared to an accepted standard or more recently, a benchmark. Standards and benchmarks are reference points that one can use to determine the quality of a programme. The institution delivering the programme or an outside agency may set standards. As previously mentioned, nursing curricula are usually reviewed by regulatory bodies for nursing or professional organizations. Accreditation is usually done by the organization and therefore the professional body sets the standards (Loriz and Foster, 2001). In addition, some form of regional standards may be set, for instance by the European Union, to enhance regional harmonization of educational standards.

Standards or benchmarks related to the following curriculum components should be explored in a holistic review. Issues of relevance, accuracy, coherence and operations are all relevant to these aspects of the curriculum. Below is a list of some components of a curriculum and what should be used as the benchmark(s).

- Programme and course outcomes – What will the graduate be able to do after qualifying?
- Course content – To achieve this, the programme will offer basic knowledge of certain critical concepts. Are those concepts included in the content? To achieve course outcomes certain lifelong learning skills are required. How is the course addressing these skills?
- Theory content hours – How much time is given for the content to be explored by the student? Is this reasonable?
- Clinical hours – In nursing, application to the real world of work is important. Are there adequate opportunities for this to be achieved?
- Clinical placement – Is the clinical setting appropriate for the learners at each level of the programme?
- Teaching strategies – Do the teaching strategies support the development of lifelong learning skills?
- Student evaluation measures – Are they appropriate in relation to the programme and course outcomes? Are there methods to ensure validity and reliability?
- Learning resources – Are they adequate and appropriate for the delivery of the programme?
- Lecturer numbers and qualifications – Are they appropriate to the programme and courses?
- Senior teaching staff qualifications, roles and responsibilities – Are they appropriate to the programme and courses?
- Administration roles and responsibilities – Do they enable the programme faculty to facilitate a positive teaching and learning experience?
- Quality assurance – Are there appropriate quality assurance mechanisms in place and are they operational?

Step two: investigating the performance or data collection

A well-planned evaluation usually defines the specific quantitative and qualitative indicators that will be used to measure whether the predetermined standards have been met and to what extent. Key to this step in the evaluation process is good leadership (Sanders, 2001). Evaluations should be planned and this includes determination of who shall take the lead in the evaluation process. Leadership may be in the form of guiding the programme team in preparation for the review, as well as guiding members of the evaluation team in the conduct of the evaluation.

Step three: synthesizing the results

Results from a review or evaluation should be compiled, analysed and widely distributed and should include conclusions and lessons learned. Findings from the evaluation, i.e., performance of the programme staff, students and graduates against a set of quantitative and qualitative criteria should be used to make judgements about the quality (fitness of purpose) of the programme. Both positive and negative findings should be shared. A focus on only those areas where weaknesses exist is demoralizing and does not emphasize the need to take advantage of those areas of programme strength.

Step four: formulating recommendations

If a developmental, improvement approach is used for the evaluation, the reviewers should very carefully consider the findings; specifically the areas where standards are not met. Clear areas for improvement should be communicated. Furthermore, in a developmental, continuous, quality-improvement approach, the evaluator(s) should provide reasonable suggestions for improvement and approaches that might be useful to alleviate or reduce deficits.

Step 5: Feeding recommendations and lessons learned back into the programme

An evaluation is only effective if it promotes improvement. This means that findings should be used in such a way that the elements of the curriculum are revised and modified, added or deleted as findings indicate. Evaluators should be able to give feedback that is critical and constructive and thus provides programme planners with information from which to develop and improve the programme further. Benchmarking or setting standards, acknowledging lessons learned (generalizations made based on several experiences) and best practices (practices that have been verified as successful in specific settings) are examples of the kinds of specific feedback that evaluators can give, especially if they are experts in the discipline, such as those involved in nursing education programme approval and accreditation.

Models of curriculum evaluation

The following section outlines some of the general information on a variety of evaluation models. The actual selection of a curriculum review or evaluation model should be based on the goals and objectives for the review or evaluation. In many cases, if the review or evaluation is a high-stakes evaluation, i.e., required for professional approval or accreditation, the model that is to be used is prescribed. If it is an internal evaluation, then the model that is selected should be one that will fulfil the evaluator's and stakeholder's expectations and requirements.

Why use a model?

Evidence suggests that the use of a model or conceptual framework for research provides direction for data collection methods and the recommendations that evolve. In evaluation research, most models include elements such as inputs (resources put into the programme prior to and during implementation), goals (what achievements the programme wishes to accomplish) and outcomes (numbers and qualities of the products of the programme). These elements provide the direction for the evaluation (Crotty, 1993).

Sarnecky (1990a) describes a four-generational structure of program evaluation models, described below.

First-generation models

First-generation models are measurement-oriented models where the evaluation is technical and based on objectively measurable data, e.g., number of students passing registration examinations or mean scores of students from a particular programme. First-generation models use measurement (usually testing of individual students) as the means of evaluation and consequently usually do not contribute to programme improvement. Furthermore, results of a first generation evaluation do not necessarily reflect the quality or appropriateness of a curriculum (Sarnecky, 1990b).

Second-generation models

Second-generation models were developed in response to the inadequacy evaluators felt using the positivist, mechanistic approach found in first-generation models (Sarnecky, 1990a). Second-generation models build on first-generation models and are characterized by their emphasis on description, specifically in relation to programme objectives. These models are a direct response to the popularity of management by objectives. In second-generation models, evaluation is based on describing how well objectives of a programme (or programme outcomes) are met. This usually includes measurement of various aspects of a programme (Sarnecky, 1990a). Tyler's (1950) model is one example of a second-generation model. Although second-generation models are broader than first-generation, the focus of these models may result in evaluation missing unintended outcomes or strengths of a programme. For this reason third generation models were developed.

Third-generation models

Third-generation models (characterized by the use of high technology) focus on using evaluation as a basis for judgement. Although most evaluations result in some kind of judgement, according to Sarneky (1990a) third-generation models make use of a wider variety of measures and description than first- and second-generation models and the focus of analysis of the data is on making judgements and planning interventions. Variations or combinations of the first three-generation models were traditionally used in evaluation for the purpose of accreditation or professional approval. In spite of the availability of useful third-generation models, it was felt that use of more qualitative, reflective methods was needed to fully understand the quality of educational programmes. The fourth-generation models were a response to this perception.

Fourth-generation models

Finally, a fourth-generation model characterized by high responsiveness has begun to evolve. In this context, responsiveness refers to the capacity of the model to enhance diagnosis of problems and achievements and make realistic judgements and recommendations based on these data. The evaluation makes use of measurement, description and judgements but goes further to look at the programme more holistically and in a more reflective manner. The responsive model is an iterative process and is characterized by negotiation, in that all elements of the programme and context are taken into consideration and inform the evaluation.

Sarnecky (1990b) describes an adapted version of Stake's model in which each of the components of the model informs the process of data collection for other components. The process, i.e., non-sequential operations, in the review is the key to the responsiveness of this adapted model. A further example of a fourth-generation model is the empowerment evaluation (Fetterman, 2002). This model is characterized by collaboration, participation and self-determination and is designed to assist programme stakeholders and to result in empowerment through self-evaluation and reflection.

Both first- and second-generation evaluation models are entrenched in a mechanistic paradigm that focuses primarily on objectively measurable elements; especially test results and achievement of objectives. Third- and fourth-generation evaluation models are a direct result of the perceived inadequacy of the first- and second-generation empirical models and are more commonly used today. Sarnecky (1990b) suggests that in order to foster dynamic, efficient programme evaluation, third- and fourth-generation models of evaluation should be employed. Additionally, responsive models of programme evaluation are the best for evaluating social or behavioural science programmes (Guba and Lincoln, 1989).

Third- and fourth-generation models are generally considered to allow for more inclusive data collection requiring a large variety of data to be collected so that the quality of data is enhanced. More holistic and comprehensive data provide a more thorough description of the issues and problems existing within a curriculum. With a more comprehensive understanding of the issues, interpretation, judgements and recommendations may be made. The depth and breadth of the data also improves the likelihood of greater validity of the evidence, depending on the methods used for the evaluation.

In the following section a brief review of the more widely used third- and fourth-generation evaluation models is provided and can be used to provide guidance in selection of an appropriate model for your curriculum review.

Review of curriculum evaluation models

CIPP

Stufflebeam's Context-Input-Process-Product (CIPP) model, formulated in the 1960s has frequently been used as a framework for evaluation of curricula (2001). As the name implies, the model includes the elements of context-input-process-products in the evaluation. In this model context refers to the type of curriculum and the objectives, input is concerned with resources required, process deals with operation and implementation and the inter-relationship between theory and practice. Product refers to the outcomes of the curriculum, in particular, the characteristics of the graduate. The model facilitates a cyclical, continuous process of evaluation and modification and can be responsive in its method of implementation. This model has proven useful for decision-making and summative evaluation in a variety of nursing curricula (e.g., Evaluation of the Diploma GN programme at the Affiliated Health Training Institutions affiliated to the University of Botswana).

Goal free

Scriven's model (1972) advocates goal-free evaluation so that achievements other than those arising from objectives can be evaluated. In this type of evaluation all outcomes are examined, not just intended outcomes, thus resulting in a highly responsive evaluation. This model can be used for decision-making and summative evaluation.

Discrepancy Evaluation

The Provus' discrepancy evaluation model is a model that searches for discrepancies between variables or elements of the curriculum, i.e., between planned and actual curriculum content, predicted and observed outcomes, student achievements and desired competencies, judgements/assessments of graduates of different groups, inconsistencies in programme objectives, content, teaching strategies, etc. (Provus, 1971). This model is useful in decision-making and summative evaluation.

Key Features

Renzulli's Key Features model suggests that evaluation should focus on the major areas of concern to the primary stakeholders. For example, the employer would be most interested in the new graduate nurses' level of competency. This model involves first determining who the stakeholder groups are and what their key features would be (Herbener and Watson, 1992). This model can be used for decision-making and both formative and summative evaluation.

Five-Step Model

The Starpoli and Waltz model specifies five steps in evaluation:

1. determine who is involved
2. state the purpose
3. identify objectives of the evaluation
4. identify evaluation activities and
5. determine when evaluation will occur.

   This model frames evaluation in terms of inputs, operations and outputs and can be responsive if implemented in a participative manner. The five-step model can be used for decision-making and formative and summative evaluations.

Countenance Model

Stake's Countenance Model suggests that description and judgement are essential elements in programme evaluation. Two matrices, a descriptive matrix and a judgement matrix, each including antecedents, transactions and outcomes, are used in this model. Antecedent refers to the conditions that exist prior to the educational intervention and can include both process and content. Examples of antecedents would be the qualifications of the faculty or the institution's admission criteria. Transactions include all the educational interventions, content and process. This component of the model could include course syllabi and teaching strategies. Outcomes include all the results of the educational innovation. Examples of outcomes would be student grades, clinical evaluations or any measurement of student achievement of terminal objectives. The model proposes that data from the description and judgement matrices are used to make decisions about the merits of a programme. This model is used for decision-making and is summative and was the first in the fourth generation of responsive models for programme evaluation (Ediger et al., 1983).

Selection of model

Selecting an evaluation model to use for review of a nursing programme is a very important step in the evaluation planning process and should occur early, ideally in the programme planning phase. The descriptions of evaluation models provided in the section above are not exhaustive but rather a beginning list of those that other evaluators of nursing programmes have found useful.

The criteria required of both the model and the evaluation tools are measurability, inclusiveness, simplicity and practicality. It is also suggested that the model selected should be based on the purpose of the evaluation, resources and needs of the programme and institution performing the evaluation. Models that focus on processes of learning, like the third- and fourth-generation models, are more likely to produce greater information on the experience and processes of learning, i.e., implementation, rather than merely outcomes of the learning (Sconce and Howard, 1994).

Conclusion

While much of the literature on evidence-based nursing practice relates to clinical practices, there is no reason why the concept cannot be used with nursing education so that standards or benchmarks are developed on the basis of evidence and efficacy of curricular models and reported experiences (lessons learned and best practices). Indeed, nurses are increasingly expected to use evidence-based practices and consumers are being given evidence-based information to improve quality of care globally (American International Health Alliance, 2003; Ellis, 2000). Curriculum adaptation and development should not be left behind in the process of using evidence to make decisions about nursing education. Therefore, benchmarking should be used in creating structures and processes that enhance quality of education. The content and processes that nursing education institutions use in educating nurses needs to contribute to the quality of care, by increasing the quality of the practitioners developed. Given the wealth of information learned from an evaluation or review, it is incumbent on nursing educators to share and apply these lessons learned and best practices in curriculum evaluation, to develop benchmarks or standards for nursing education.

Development of a database of benchmarks for nursing education would be a very worthwhile exercise as there is a dearth of empirical evidence of what practices are 'best practices' and in what context they are most likely to be effective. Benchmarking research in this area using data from review and evaluation would advance knowledge in the area of nursing education as well as the science of evaluation.

Evaluation of nursing education is a professional responsibility and should be approached in a systematic, collegial fashion. In this chapter the definitions, purpose, types and steps of evaluation are followed by an introduction to several common curriculum evaluation models. This brief overview of curriculum evaluation is provided in order to advance the quality of nursing programmes globally.

Points for discussion

1. Which model do you like best? Why?
2. What influence would the model you selected have on the preparation for evaluation?
3. What do you think are the strengths and weaknesses in your programme? Why?
4. What would you recommend to improve your programme, i.e., maximize strengths or reduce weaknesses?

References

American International Health Alliance (2003) Learning Resource Center Project: Practice Standards Reviews. Online. HTTP: http://www.aiha.com (accessed 26 January 2005).

Chevasse, J. (1994) Curriculum evaluation in nursing education: a review of the literature. *Journal of Advanced Nursing,* 19: 1024–1031.

Crotty, M. (1993) Curriculum issues related to the newly developed nursing diploma courses. *Nurse Education Today,* 13: 264–269.

Ediger, J., Snyder, M. and Corcoran, S. (1983) Selecting a model for use in curriculum evaluation. *Journal of Nursing Education,* 22(5): 195–199.

Ellis, J. (2000) Sharing the evidence: Clinical practice benchmarking to improve continuously the quality of care. *Journal of Advanced Nursing,* 32(2): 215–225.

Fetterman, D. M. (2002) *Foundations of Empowerment Evaluation.* Thousand Oaks, CA: Sage.

Gerbic, P. and Kranenburg, I. (2003) The impact of external approval processes on programme development. *Quality in Higher Education,* 9(2): 169–177.

Gilroy, P., Long, P., Rangecroft, M. and Tricker, T. (2001) Evaluation and the invisible student: theories, practice and problems in evaluating distance education. *Quality Assurance in Education,* 9(1): 14–22.

Guba, E. and Lincoln, Y.S. (1989) *Fourth Generation Evaluation.* San Francisco, CA: Jossey Bass.

Herbener, D. J. and Watson, J. E. (1992) Models of evaluating nursing education programs. *Nursing Outlook,* 40(1): 27–32.

Hopkin, A. G. (2003). *Frame Factors and a Quality Assurance Agency in a Developmental Context. Proceedings Seventh Biennial Conference of the International Network of Quality Assurance Agencies in Higher Education: A Regional Perspective.* Dublin, Ireland.

Loriz L. M. and Foster, P. H. (2001) Focus groups: Powerful adjuncts for program evaluation. *Nursing Forum,* 36(3): 31–36.

Lusky, M. B. and Hayes, R. L. (2001). Collaborative consultation and program evaluation. *Journal of Counseling & Development,* 79: 26–38.

Perry, J. C. (2001) Enhancing instructional programs through evaluation: Translating theory into practice. *Community College Journal of Research and Practice*, **25**: 573–590.

Priest, S. (2001) A program evaluation primer. *The Journal of Experiential Education*, **24**(1): 34–40.

Prosavac, E. J. and Carey, R. G. (1997) *Program Evaluation: Methods and Case Studies*, 3rd edn. New Jersey: Prentice Hall.

Provus, M. (1971) *Discrepancy Evaluation*. Berkeley: McCutchan.

Sanders, J. R. (2001) A vision for evaluation. *American Journals of Evaluation* **22**(3): 363–366.

Sarnecky, M. T. (1990a) Program evaluation. Part 1: Four generations of theory. *Nurse Educator*, **15**(5): 25–28.

Sarnecky, M. T. (1990b) Program evaluation. Part 1: Four generations of theory. *Nurse Educator*, **15**(6): 7–10.

Scone, C. and Howard, J. (1994) Curriculum evaluation: A new approach. *Nurse Education Today*, **14**(4): 280–286.

Scriven, M. S. (1972). The methodology of evaluation, in P. A. Taylor and D. M. Cowley (eds.) *Readings in Curriculum Evaluation*. Dubuque, IO: Wm. C. Brown Company Publishers.

Stufflebeam, D. L. (2001) *Evaluation Models*. New York: John Wiley & Sons.

Sutcliffe, L. (1992) An examination of the implications of adopting a process approach to curriculum planning, implementation and evaluation. *Journal of Advanced Nursing*, **17**: 1496–1502.

Thomas, B., Rajacich, D., Al Ma'aitah, R., Cameron, S. J. and Malinowski, A. (2000) Advancing the development of human resources in nursing in Jordan. *Journal of Continuing Education in Nursing*, **31**(3): 135–140.

Thomas, B, Rajacich, D., Al Ma'aitah, R., Cameron, S. J., Gharaibeh, M. and Delahunt, T. D. (2002). Developing a programme review process for a baccalaureate nursing programme in Jordan. *International Nursing Review*, **47**: 243–247.

Tyler, R.W. (1950) *Basic Principles of Curriculum and Instructions*. Chicago, IL: University of Chicago Press.

UNFPA (2001) *Monitoring and Evaluation Toolkit for Programme Managers. Tool No. 1*. Online available at: www.unfpa.org/monitoring/toolkit.

Recommended reading

Lee, M.B., Sumar, F., Beaton, S. and Marshall, P. (2001) Working Paper 01–05 *Evaluation of Implementation of Basic RN Revised Curriculum – Year I*. Ontario: University of Toronto-McMaster University Press.

This paper gives an example of the use of a fourth generation model to evaluate a curriculum.

Fishman, D.B. and Neigher, W.D. (2003) Publishing systematic, pragmatic case studies in program evaluation: rationale and introduction to the special issue. *Evaluation and Program Planning*, **26**(4), 421–428.

Further examples of curriculum evaluation are described in this article.

Lynch, D.C., Greer, A.G., Larson, L.C., Cummings, D.M., Harriett, B.S., Dreyfus, K.S. and Clay, M.C. (2003) Descriptive metaevaluation: case study of an interdisciplinary curriculum. *Evaluation & the Health Professions,* **26**(4), 447–461.

This final example deals with the evaluation of a multidisciplinary curriculum.

Helpful URLs for further study:

http://www.ieq.org/Tools/index.htm

http://www.qaa.ac.uk/

http://www.aiha.com

http://www.gonzaga.edu/rap/

Chapter 8

A problem-based learning curriculum

Henry Y Akinsola

Introduction

Problem-based learning (PBL) has a long tradition of specialized instruction in post-secondary academic institutions, especially medical, nursing and allied health education (Berkson, 1993; Bruhn, 1997). PBL can be defined as an approach to learning and instruction in which students tackle problems in small groups under the supervision of a teacher. In this context, a problem consists of the description of a set of phenomena or events that can be perceived in reality. These phenomena have to be analysed or explained by the tutorial group in terms of underlying principles, mechanisms or processes. The tools used in order to do that are discussion of the problem and studying relevant resources (Schmidt, 1993). According to Bruhn (1997), PBL occurs when students are put in a task environment that allows them to carry out all the cognitive steps that would represent a real-life situation. Students are prompted by teachers to learn what they need to know in order to solve the problem. Their own questions become hypotheses, prompting more inquiry and questions. Students develop critical reasoning processes and an appreciation of the range of information needed to answer their questions and how the information is interrelated. What is important to emphasize, however, is that PBL is only a strategy and that teachers must define their objectives and expected outcomes (Norman and Schmidt, 1992).

Characteristics of PBL

The essential elements of PBL are a strong focus on the process of learning, the teacher as a guide to learning or a facilitator of learning, learning in context facilitates retrieval of information, and learning is the responsibility of the learner.

A strong focus on the process of learning

PBL is a process-oriented curriculum, which defines the process that will be used for learning and constructs the curriculum so that this process is central to all learning experiences. The philosophy that underpins a process-oriented curriculum suggests that learning is a process and knowledge is constructed rather than merely acquired. Process-oriented does not mean that the programme has no specific or essential content; indeed, problem-based curricula are very specific in defining the concepts that are essential to an educational programme. For example in McMaster University all nursing courses taught through problems-based small group tutorials, have syllabi that outline the concepts that will be explored during the course. The problem scenarios are constructed to facilitate exploration of these concepts. In the author's experience, making this information explicit and sharing this information with learners is essential to satisfaction and confidence in the process for both teaching staff and students. Frequently students need reassurance that they are 'learning the right thing' and learning at an appropriate level. Informing students of the deliberate construction of problem-based scenarios enhances student trust in the process.

Process-oriented means that the teaching staff are committed to the notion that the key to learning fundamental concepts is through a systematic process. The teaching staff who implement the curriculum must be convinced that if essential concepts are 'embedded' in the context of a problem, students will acquire the relevant knowledge. Philosophically, the programme-teaching staff must be convinced or converted to it, if that is what is required of the idea that if the problem-solving process is used to its optimum the student will discover and construct essential knowledge (content). Without this philosophical position the problem-solving process, as well as the construction of problem scenarios, is likely to be impaired.

The teacher is a guide to learning or a facilitator of learning

With the commitment to a process-oriented curriculum comes a dramatic shift in the role of the teaching staff. The role of knowledge transmitter is no longer appropriate but must transform to facilitator in the use and development of problem-solving skills. The philosophy pertaining to the role of a teacher must shift from what Durgahee (1988), calls a 'sage on stage' to a 'guide on the side'. In PBL, learners determine the goals of the educational encounter and they are guided in the most efficient means of gathering and constructing knowledge to achieve these goals. The commitment of teaching staff to guiding rather than transmitting knowledge is a fundamental philosophical foundation. The mandate for teaching staff to guide rather than transmit knowledge is generally true in process-oriented curricula but is particularly true for problem-based curricula because teaching/learning situations often occur in small groups with teachers acting as facilitators rather than vessels of wisdom. Because this process of education is relatively new, teachers have little training and/or development in the techniques for this teaching/learning strategy. The result can be that when a difficult situation arises teachers return to the behaviours that they are most comfortable with and the classroom becomes the vehicle for transmission of teachers' knowledge rather than learners' opportunity to develop inquiry skills to create and discover knowledge.

Unfortunately, it is not only teachers who are sometimes uncomfortable with this role transition. Learners must also be enlightened and transformed. Students must alter their educational expectations. Because students' educational experience has been primarily with traditional teacher-centred approaches, learners are reluctant to assume greater control over their learning environment. It is not uncommon for students to object initially to a new approach. This phenomenon highlights the importance of (a) a strong philosophical foundation for the programme, (b) undivided commitment by teaching staff, and (c) appropriate orientation of the learners to the philosophy of the programme.

Learning in context facilitates retrieval of information

Significant research has been conducted that supports the value of contextualized, integrated learning and its role in knowledge development and retrieval (Amos and White, 1998; Biley and Smith, 1998). Most studies on the efficacy of PBL have been performed with medical students. These studies have demonstrated that knowledge that is presented contextually promotes storage of information in a way that facilitates rapid retrieval of information (Albanese and Mitchell, 1993). PBL forces learners to encounter information and problems in context or real-life situations. With the contextualization of problems, professional practice knowledge becomes part of long-term memory and can be used in a variety of real life problem situations. Students can be guided to learn in this manner and as a result will store information for future use that can be applied in professional practice. The difference between the novice and the expert is this ability to translate what one has learned or experienced before to a new situation (Benner, 1984). It is likely that PBL is one approach that can be used to reduce the theory–practice gap and facilitate the progression from novice to expert. Learning in context enables students to organize their long-term memory for ready retrieval (Schmidt, 1993). PBL encourages effectiveness of the application of different forms of knowledge and the understanding of various concepts in such a way as to clarify pertinent factors and their interactions and interconnectedness.

Learning is the responsibility of the learner

The philosophic view that the learner is responsible for his/her own learning is essential to the success of problem-based learning. Without this philosophical view teaching staff have difficulty in fostering students' problem-solving. The shift in perspective to student responsibility for learning is particularly difficult for educators who are familiar and comfortable with teacher-directed learning. A significant reason for these educators' discomfort is the loss of teacher control in the classroom. The feeling of loss of control comes with sharing the 'stage' with the learners (Durgahee, 1988).

The view that a teacher can force or even facilitate learning when learners are not motivated and do not accept responsibility for their learning is inconsistent with the philosophic underpinnings of problem-based learning. This view reverts to the traditional role of the teacher who has all the knowledge and has only to transmit this knowledge and it will be learned, a view totally inconsistent with PBL philosophical foundations. As mentioned previously, students also need to be guided in transforming their views of education. Without full understanding of the philosophy and the support of a committed teaching staff students will reject their responsibility for learning.

The rationale for PBL

In most higher education institutions today, including the universities that offer nursing programmes, the main feature seems to be large groups of students under the authority of a teacher who orally transmits information to them on a particular discipline. In these settings, the students are in a passive situation, their only activity being to take notes. Traditionally, such institutions expect the teachers to assess the performance of the students and not to verify the quality of the teaching/learning process. Heliker (1994) from her experience as clinical faculty for baccalaureate nursing students, maintains that basic science knowledge acquired in the classroom, such as pharmacology, are not always retained and transferred to the practice setting. When faced with real patients and medications in the clinical setting, she observed that students were often unable to relate the cold facts of 'knowing that' with the interpersonal, contextual 'knowing how'. Kimmel (1992) also observed similar difficulties when teaching pathophysiology to second year medical students, leading him to abandon the lecture format.

French (1992) conducted an analysis of British literature from 1961 to 1982 and found that in Britain, the educational paradigm over the past decade was teacher-centred, with the student being the passive recipient of information. French (1992) contends that the outcome of learning failed to exhibit a patient-oriented, critically thinking individual, capable of adequate decision-making in practice.

Advances in science, computer and medical technology are expanding the scope of health knowledge at an ever-increasing pace so that it is no longer possible to teach everything or learn everything. Students therefore need to learn how to learn what they need in order to deal with personal and professional problems as they appear. It is also noteworthy, that just like the health system, the other sectors within the national service, such as education and industry have also experienced exponential growth. The higher literacy rate and improved socio-economic standard of the people led to the creation of greater awareness of their right, including the right to receive adequate nursing care and for higher education students to receive high quality education.

To meet these challenges, the role of educators is to encourage students to find and make effective use of the resources which they need to carry out their professional tasks in all practice settings. Therefore, the aim to be achieved is to help students in the course of their training to become the architects of their own education, which will enable them to cope with learning as a lifelong event (Bruhn, 1997; Vernon and Blake, 1993). In such a situation, there is need for teachers to orientate themselves in such a way that they resist the temptation of seeing themselves as the custodians of knowledge. Instead, the role of educators should be the planning of learning activities so as to give students the opportunity to be proactive in their learning.

International literature over a period of 20 years reviewed by Albanese and Mitchell (1993) and Vernon and Blake (1993) concluded that PBL is judged by students and faculty to be effective as shown by the following findings: it appears to be favoured over other styles of learning, to be efficient and to accomplish its objectives.

Norman and Schmidt (1992) carried out an extensive review of literature on studies, which address different aspects of the evaluation of PBL. In spite of the variation in the results of the reviewed studies, the conclusion was that a PBL curriculum facilitates long-term memory retrieval, may encourage integration of learned concepts to new clinical situations, and enhances the development of long-lasting self-directed learning skills. Furthermore, different authors also reported that PBL medical students use more resources and are more self-directed than their non-PBL counterparts (Blumberg and Michael, 1992; Sanders et al., 1985). William et al. (1993) showed that PBL graduates appear to have broader social and interpersonal skills, a greater appreciation of the complexity of problems and the resources available for solution and a heightened motivation for continued self-learning. Most authors therefore conclude that students who graduate from a PBL curriculum are more likely to be better prepared for practice than those from a 'traditional curriculum'.

With specific reference to nursing education, PBL seems to have a number of advantages, according to Helicker (1994). This approach enhances the problem-solving capability and the acquisition of such nursing skills as the logical approach and self-directed learning, it facilitates learning team collaboration, learning to listen and participate in interdisciplinary discussion. Furthermore, students become socialized as colleagues and professionals and each of them learns not only to value his/her own ways of knowing, but to obtain and accept information from various other sources, to question others critically and to obtain feedback on his/her own learning outcome.

In spite of the numerous advantages of the PBL approach, it is worthy of note that it also has some disadvantages, as follows:

- The requirements of PBL are very demanding for both the teachers and students. As an innovative approach, which is quite different from the traditional method, it demands a different mind-set regarding the learning objectives, the learning process and methods of evaluation or assessments.

- Another disadvantage of the method with respect to some countries is that the adoption of the PBL approach by any institution requires total commitment to two things:
  - Reorientation of the institutional philosophy to embrace the PBL model for curriculum development and implementation of programmes. This has proved difficult in many institutions because of the resistance to change by policymakers and managers of academic programmes, such as deans of faculties and heads of departments.
  - Provision of additional resources or redistribution of existing ones to facilitate student-directed learning (which is a major component of PBL) through unlimited access to information. To guarantee the success of programmes based on the PBL model, the library, the computer services, the audio-visual aid facilities, laboratories, classroom spaces, clinical facilities and community setting must be adequate.

Developing a PBL curriculum

The concepts teaching and learning are often used interchangeably and educators tend to take for granted that teaching would lead to learning. Van der Vleuten et al. (1996) point out that although educators almost automatically talk about their programmes in terms of teaching, education is essentially about learning. In educational change, this aspect (learning) should be the focus of attention, since teaching is only the instrument towards learning.

The significance of the above paragraph is that PBL is a learning programme rather than a teaching programme. In the PBL process, the centre of the universe is the student. It is based on the idea of self-directed learning (SDL), which is an important vehicle in PBL. Instead of delivering lectures, tutors (lecturers) give an overview of the topic and when necessary, clarify difficult concepts. Students learn as individuals and as peer groups rather than attend lectures. The lecture halls are replaced by the library and learning facilities. Furthermore, the long hours of the end of year examination should be replaced by a gradual process of continuous assessment, which helps students to use information to understand phenomena or problems and to apply knowledge to relevant context instead of displaying it.

The process of adopting the PBL model by a faculty and implementing the curriculum can be categorized into four areas. From the discussion of the different steps and processes that follow, it will become evident that each of the stages is not mutually exclusive. In other words, the process is dynamic and it includes the following:

Faculty commitment and development

Experience has shown that in any institution intending to adopt a PBL model, the first and perhaps one of the most important processes takes place at a point when an individual or group shows an appreciation for the need for change in the traditional educational method and moves a step forward to initiate the change, i.e. readiness to serve as a change agent. This calls for the commitment of the authority of the institution, most especially the head of the school, or dean of the faculty. The whole faculty must show commitment to the plan right from the onset. Therefore, both the institutional philosophy, the mission statement and programme objectives must as a sine qua non clearly show commitment to adopting the model and indicating the direction for curriculum development and programme implementation. The faculty as a team must adjust their attitude regarding the goals of nursing education and the methods of achieving these goals.

Resource development and allocation

By resource, the author refers to both human and other resources. One of the greatest challenges facing the adopters of the PBL approach, especially the authority or programme managers, is provision and management of resources. There must be enough resources to achieve the objectives of the programme. Since teaching is kept to the barest minimum, students need to have access to both the print and electronic media and other learning resources, such as up-to-date text books, periodicals, video-tapes, audio-cassettes, anatomical models and charts, good laboratories, tutorial classes, clinical sites (both in the community and hospitals), as well as human resources, such as tutors, technologists/technicians, demonstrators and other support staff. In order to achieve this mission, enough resources need to be dedicated to allow the faculty to be creative and to test relevant models of PBL both in the institution and the community. This does not necessarily imply that old resources should be discarded in order to bring in new ones but all could be reorganized together to ensure prudent management of available resources.

As regards human resource development, once the commitments have been firmly secured, the members of the faculty, comprising both the academic and non-academic staff, must be orientated in such a way that they can adjust to the demands and challenges of the new approach. For example, in the Faculty of Health Sciences, Moi University, Eldoret, Kenya, each member of both the academic and technical staff underwent a training programme which took the form of a workshop for 3–4 days. Once the programme was implemented, new staff were not allowed to participate in PBL without such training. The workshop helps participants to acquire new knowledge and skills in different aspects of the programme, such as how to develop cases, conduct tutorials, give course overviews, provide mentorship to students, and students' assessment. After the workshop, new members of staff are usually teamed up with more experienced members and they then progress from observing tutorial sessions to facilitating them.

The continuing education programme in the faculty was tailored towards helping the staff to update their knowledge and skill regularly, accommodate/ assimilate other views of learning and develop the prerequisite PBL pedagogy (teaching skill) which according to Creedy et al. (1992) includes the following five principles:

1.   an awareness of one's own beliefs about teaching and learning
2.   a conceptual change in teaching approach
3.   the ability to focus
4.   negotiations
5.   analysis of students' learning.

Curriculum development

According to Swanson et al. (1991), there are two types of PBL curricula: an open discovery and a guided discovery approach. The open discovery approach emphasizes that students should have the responsibility for determining what, when and how to learn. Students learn to apply broad principles during group sessions with minimum guidance from the tutors. This, they believe, leads to maximal opportunity for exploration by students and for initiation of lifelong learning. In contrast to the open discovery method, in the guided discovery method curriculum designers for each problem identify specific learning objectives. The objectives are provided to the tutors who use them to organize group discussions and other learning experiences. This is the approach usually used in health professional education.

The design of a PBL curriculum, as in the case of the traditional method, is guided by the philosophy, the objectives and the conceptual framework adopted by the faculty. Hence, most of the processes involved in developing a PBL curriculum have already been dealt with in the preceding chapters dealing with the process of curriculum development, especially the chapter on developing a macro-curriculum. This section therefore, highlights those processes which differentiate the PBL curriculum development process from that of developing a traditional curriculum.

A multidisciplinary curriculum committee

In designing a PBL curriculum the need to ensure that the curriculum development committee is multidisciplinary in its constitution cannot be over emphasized. This ensures that the problem scenarios are well integrated and have a broad disciplinary focus as would be encountered in the clinical context. For instance, a biochemist will bring important but different information from that which would be obtained from a social scientist. Within the nursing discipline itself, a mental health nurse brings to the problem development a different perspective from that of a community health nurse or a general nurse.

Identification and selection of health problems for inclusion in the curriculum

The source of problems to be dealt with must be the authentic clinical situations that the learners are most likely to encounter. Decisions to include specific health problems in a PBL curriculum should be based on what are currently the most common conditions, their impact on the health status of the community and/or nation and potential for nursing intervention. Problems which are exotic, with little potential for nursing intervention, may be interesting to know but have really no place in a PBL curriculum. Learning through PBL is slow and demands all the time that an education institution has with the students, so emphasis must fall on common, realistic problems.

Developing a concept map for problem development

Once the health problems have been identified, an outline of the main concepts around which the problem scenarios is developed must be constructed. Such a conceptual outline is essential to make sure that the curriculum does not revert to disease orientation without much opportunity for integration during the learning process. Such a concept outline may include broad concepts such as immobility, fever, pain, poverty, etc.

Deciding on the number, focus and organization of problem scenarios for each identified broad concept

Some concepts may be so broad that more than one problem scenario might be necessary in order to treat them effectively within a nursing curriculum. For instance the committee needs to decide whether the basic sciences (biomedical and social sciences) that need to be learned in relation to immobility might be better learned in a separate problem scenario from that dealing with clinical (nursing) management of health problems associated with immobility. This part of the process requires that clear learning objectives be defined for each identified major concept. Decisions about organizational structure of the curriculum, with regard to sequencing and continuity (vertical relationships) and integration (horizontal relationships) should be congruent with the nursing school's articulated philosophy and conceptual framework for nursing and nursing education.

Problem scenario development

Problem scenario development for the PBL approach poses a great challenge to tutors or nurse educators. To meet this challenge, problem scenarios should be developed for each course within each of the disciplines (e.g. anatomy) by an interdisciplinary team of the nursing school faculty. Each scenario is then presented to the entire faculty for review and approval. It is of paramount importance that each scenario should help students to achieve the key learning objective for a particular course. For each course, a case booklet, commonly known as a problem package, should be produced. A booklet consists of all the problem scenarios, the exercises and illustrations/diagrams. Apart from the course booklet, another booklet is prepared which is referred to as a tutors' guide. This second booklet is exclusively for the use of the tutors because it contains the list of what the students are expected to achieve in each of their tutorial groups, after discussing and analysing each case. A list of resources is optional as there are those who believed that PBL students should locate these resources themselves (Drummond-Young and Mohide, 2001).

Most schools, however, generally have one problem package to which only the facilitator has access, and which is kept in a central bank. The main components of the problem package include a problem scenario, patient and/or client data, tutor's guide and if desired a list of resources (Drummond-Young and Mohide, 2001). See Chapter 12 for a detailed description of the problem scenario development process.

The tutorial process in PBL

The heart of the PBL approach is the meeting of the tutorial group. During tutorials, students review/study and analyse the cases/problems in small groups of 6–8. Each small group uses the problem to ensure a meaningful context to learning. As was previously mentioned, by providing this context, knowledge can be integrated with previous knowledge and knowledge can be better retrieved when necessary.

In the context of a tutorial class, a problem can be defined as the (more or less neutral) description of a certain number of phenomena or events, which appear to be related in certain ways. In the group the students first analyse the phenomena, and then gradually work out a plan of action to resolve the problem and acquire the necessary skills to implement the plan. Problems cover a wide range of issues, not just practical skills or individual client problems.

Although the process of a tutorial is generally the same in all the institutions where PBL curricula are being implemented, there is no standard procedure for initiating and sustaining the process of learning. It should be stressed that the process of orientation of students to the method and process of learning is very important. For example, Brandon and Majumdar (1997) explained that in their school, on the first day of class, students were oriented to the PBL approach through a 2.5-hour class session devoted to completing an interactive study guide, viewing a 60-minute video tape and participating in a practice session. The video introduced the first case problem to be used in the course. During this orientation activity, students took turns facilitating the group process and recording the hypothesis and learning issues developed during the process.

Also in the faculty of Health Sciences, Moi University, Eldoret, Kenya, the department known as the Department of Medical Education is charged with the responsibility of conducting orientation programmes for both new students and staff. This department runs a one-unit course, which is titled: 'Basics of Medical Education'. The objectives of the course are as follows:

1. Explain the philosophy and objectives of the Faculty of Health sciences.
2. Describe the design and implementation of the degree programme (Medicine, Environmental Health Science or Nursing Science).
3. Compare and contrast traditional and innovative teaching/learning methods in Medical Education.
4. Describe the roles of tutors and students in PBL.
5. State various assessment methods and tests used in Medical Education.

Whatever system of PBL is adopted by an educational institution, four distinct phases are noticeable in the PBL process: the initial encounter with the problem, self-directed learning activities (SDL), subsequent encounter with the problem, and attaining problem closure. In general, each tutorial group meets twice a week for about 1–2 hours per session. During the first tutorial class, the group selects the chairperson and rapporteur by consensus. The chairperson controls the group's activities while the rapporteur/secretary keeps minutes on the board. Both positions are rotated among the members of the group after every session. Table 8.1 presents a synopsis of the four phases of the PBL process.

Initial encounter with the problem

The initial encounter with the problem constitutes the students' initial introduction to what they are expected to learn. This means that, instead of the usual topic outlines and/or learning objectives, the students meet 'the patient' first, rather than content or objectives. During this initial encounter with the problem, learners are expected to: (a) clarify the terms and concepts, (b) formulate the problem and identify its components, (c) suggest possible explanations, (d) conduct assessment through inquiry or data collection, (e) schematize and classify the hypotheses derived in step (c), and (f) identify learning issues (i.e. formulate enabling educational objectives).

Table 8.1 The tutorial process

---

1. Initial encounter with the problem: problem formulation
   1.1. Clarify terms and concepts
   1.2. Formulate the problem and identify its components
   1.3. Suggest possible explanations
   1.4. Collect data
   1.5. Schematize and classify the hypotheses in step 3
   1.6. Formalize and select learning issues

2. Self-directed learning activities
   2.1. Locating and consulting learning resources outside the classroom
   2.2. Reading and interpreting text in the light of the problem
   2.3. Questioning and verifying own understanding with relevant human resources
        (subject experts, patients, and/or relatives, policymakers, etc.)

3. Subsequent encounter with the problem: synthesis and review of newly acquired information
   3.1. Formulate most likely explanation
   3.2. Propose what action should or would be taken
   3.3. Carry out action where feasible or appropriate
   3.4. Verify effectiveness of action

4. Attaining problem closure
   4.1. Formulate further study questions
   4.2. Review group process and progress

Adapted from Guilbert, 1987.

The initial session is spent getting to know the 'patient' with the presenting problem, through a process of brainstorming and questioning by both the students and the facilitator. A number of plausible explanations regarding what could possibly be 'wrong' with the patient, as well as the underlying causes of the problem, are explored.

Students are expected to ask for any information they need in order to understand the problem, however such information should not require the facilitator to guess. It should be information that would normally be acquired through assessment (individual, family or community – depending on the nature of the problem). As the students get more patient or client (family or community) data through assessment, they begin to eliminate those hypotheses that no longer seem plausible in the light of information they now have, which they did not have before. The first encounter ends with students identifying areas on which they need more information – commonly referred to as 'learning issues' in a PBL session. Usually students divide the learning issues among the group. It is important, however, to stress that it is more conducive to the group process to read more than the allocated or selected learning issues so as to be able to participate in the whole discussion with some insight into what other group members are talking about.

The discussion affords students space to validate their understanding of what they learned regarding the problem through discussion with colleagues, a process which cognitive learning psychologists refer to as elaboration. Elaboration of information enhances understanding and processing of information for storage in long-term memory. Students benefit from elaboration when they explain what they have learned rather than when listening to others present what they have learned. Hence, it is important that all the students in the group participate in group discussion – i.e. get an opportunity to 'elaborate' on what they have learned (McCown et al., 1996).

Self-directed learning activities

Having identified what they need to learn, the students are now on their own. Students should be encouraged to look beyond textual resources. A list of subject experts is usually provided to the facilitator as part of the problem package. This information is only given to students on request. It is not volunteered by the facilitator.

After identifying the learning issues, the tutorial group breaks up and so the learning objectives or identified issues become homework assignments, which they have to complete through SDL before the next tutorial. Usually, there is an interval of about 3–4 days (e.g. Mondays and Thursdays of every week). At the next tutorial session, group members discuss what they have found in a manner that demonstrates understanding of the problem or the identified issues (and not by reading out notes). That SDL experience which usually takes place during the few days between the first and the second tutorials helps students to expand their knowledge about the learning objectives and to re-examine the identified issues or problems in the light of new information. In other words, students begin to change or modify their views/hypothesis about the problem, based on the acquired knowledge.

In PBL, self-directed learning, however, is not an event but a process. Throughout the tutorial process, through cognitive modeling the facilitator guides the students through the process of monitoring their own learning, identifying gaps in knowledge as well as ineffective thinking processes.

Subsequent encounter with the problem

During discussions in subsequent meetings of the group with their tutor, i.e. during the next tutorial, the completeness of the learning process, with respect to the learning objectives and the correctness of what has been learned are ascertained and evaluated. At this point of encounter with the problem, it is expected that students now know more about the problem than they did at the end of the first encounter. Hence, it is important for the facilitator to ascertain what resources were used. Students are taught, through questioning, the skill of judging the credibility of the sources they use. For instance, how old is the source? What is the frame of reference of the author? Would authors writing from different frames of reference have arrived at the same conclusion about this particular problem? Such questions help learners understand and appreciate the contextual and historical nature of most human knowledge.

The session focuses on the application of new knowledge to the problem. Through inquiry and analysis of prior decisions and/or inferences in the light of new knowledge, students begin the process of validating and/or refuting some of the hypotheses generated during the initial encounter with the problem (Barrows, 1988).

When the students are left with only what they believe to be the most likely explanation, a plan of action is proposed, and carried out where appropriate or feasible.

Attaining problem closure

This is one of the essential components of the PBL process. It is the facilitator's responsibility to ensure that students attain closure on the problem. Through questioning and guidance, he/she needs to ensure that the students are able to pull together all the information learned during the initial session, SDL activities and the subsequent session. Before the problem is closed, both the facilitator and the learners must be clear as to exactly what the focus of the problem was, what possible nursing interventions could be applied and to what purpose. At this stage of the learning process if there are outstanding issues, new objectives must be set and these become homework assignments, which should be dealt with during the first tutorial of the following week.

Hence attaining closure includes formulating further study questions as well as assessing the group process with regard to progress toward achieving learning outcomes. The review should conclude with feedback from individuals, the group, peers and the tutor. The feedback should show how well each member contributed to the group process, what other members could do to improve their performance and how the overall learning process could be improved.

Conclusion

The role of nurse–educator should be to create a flexible learning environment through the application of educational strategies, such as PBL, which focus on eliciting students' concepts and reasoning processes through SDL, group facilitation and negotiation skills. Unlike the traditional nursing curricula, which often create stressors for both students and teachers, in PBL programmes, students have pleasure in studying and are more motivated. In fact students view PBL learning as 'fun'. This approach seems to hold promise for nursing in the new millennium.

Points for discussion

1. How can we make sure the nursing students cover all the content they need if a PBL curriculum is used?
2. Is such a radical change (from traditional to PBL) really necessary?

References

Albanese, M. and Mitchell, S, (1993) Problem-based learning: a review of literature on its outcome and implementation issues. *Academic Medicine* **68**(1): 52– 81.

Amos, E. and White, M. J. (1998). Teaching tools: Problem-based learning. *Nurse Educator*, **23**(2), 11–14, 21.

Barrows, H. (1988) *The Tutorial Process*. Springfield, Illinois: Southern Illinois School of Medicine.

Benner, P. (1984) *From Novice to Expert*. Menlo Park, CA: Addison Wesley.

Berkson, L. (1993) Problem-based learning: have expectations been met? *Academic Medicine*, **68**(suppl. 10): 579–588.

Biley, F. C. and Smith, K. L. (1998). Exploring the potential of problem-based learning in nurse education. *Nurse Education Today*, **18**: 353–361.

Blumberg, P. and Michael, J. (1992) Development of self-directed learning behaviour in a partially teacher directed problem based learning curriculum. *Teaching and Learning in Medicine* **4**(1): 3–8.

Brandon, J. E. and Majumdar, B. (1997) An introduction and evaluation of problem based learning in health profession education. *Family Community Health*; **20**(1): 1–15.

Bruhn, J. G. (1997) Outcomes of problem-based learning in health care professional education: A critique. *Family Community Health*, **20**(1): 66–74.

Creedy, D., Horsfall, J. and Hand, B. (1992) Problem-based learning in nurse education: an Australian view. *Journal of Advanced Nursing*, **17**: 727–733.

Drummond-Young, M. and Mohide, E. A. (2001) Developing problems for use in problem-based learning. In E. Rideout (ed.) *Transforming Nursing Education through Problem-based Learning*. Toronto, Canada: Jones and Bartlett.

Durgahee, T. (1988) Facilitating reflection: from a sageon stage to a guide on the side. *Nurse Education Today*, **18**: 158–164.

French, P. (1992) The quality of nurse education in the 1980s. *Journal of Advanced Nursing*, **17**: 619–631.

Guilbert, J. J. (1987) *Educational Handbook for Health Personnel*, 6th edn. WHO Offset Publication No 35. Geneva: WHO.

Helicker, D. (1994) Meeting the challenge of the curriculum revolution. Problem-based learning in nursing education. *Journal of Nursing Education*, **33**(1): 45–47.

Kimmel, P. (1992) Abandoning the lecture: Curriculum reform in the introduction to clinical medicine. *The Pharos*, **Spring**: 36–71.

McCown, R., Driscoll, M. and Roop, P. G. (1996) *Educational Psychology: A Learning Centered Approach to Classroom Practice*. Boston, MA: Allyn and Bacon.

Moi University (1995) Curriculum for the Bachelor of Medicine and Bachelor of Surgery (M.B., Ch.B.), Faculty of Health Sciences. Eldoret, Kenya: Moi University.

Norman, G. T. and Schmidt, H. G. (1992) The psychological basis of problem-based learning: a review of evidence. *Academic Medicine*, **67**: 557–565.

Sanders, K., Northup, D. and Mennin, S. (1985) The library in a problem-based curriculum. In: Kaufmanis, A. (ed) *Implementing Problem-Based Medical Education: Lessons from Successful Innovations*. New York: Springer.

Schmidt, H. G. (1993) Foundations of problem-based learning: some explanatory notes. *Medical Education*, **27**: 422–432.

Swanson, D., Case, S., van der Vleuten, C. P. M. (1991). Strategies for student assessment. In D. Boud and G. Felletti (eds) *The Challenge of Problem-Based Learning*. London: Kogan Page.

Van Der Vleuten, C. P. M, Scerpbier, W.H.F.W. and Snellen, H.A.M. (1996) Flexibility in learning: a case report on problem based learning. *International Higher Education*, Second Issue, 17–24.

Vernon, D. T. A. and Blake, R. L. (1993) Does problem-based learning work? A meta-analysis of evaluative research. *Academic Medicine*, **68**: 550–563.

William, R., Saarinen-Rahikka H. and Norman, G. R. (1993) Self directed learning in problem-based health sciences education. *Academic Medicine*, **68**: 161–163.

Recommended reading

Iputo, J. E. (1999) Impact of the problem-based learning curriculum on the learning styles and strategies of medical students at the University of Transkei. *SA Medical Journal*, **89**(5): 550–554.

This article describes how the learning styles and strategies of 132 medical students were monitored over the 4 years of a PBL medical curriculum, using the Lancaster Inventory on Study Strategies. It showed a significant improvement in a number of variables, such as decreasing examination fear, and increasing versatile and operational learning.

Uys, L. R., Gwele, N. S., McInerney, P., Van Rhyn, L. L. and Tanga, T. T. (2004) The competence of nursing graduates from problem-based programmes in South Africa. *Journal of Nursing Education*, **43**(8): 352–361.

This article describes a qualitative study, based on Benner's stages of practice, comparing the competence of graduates of four PBL programmes with graduates of traditional programmes 6 months after graduation. Most graduates described incidents at levels ranging from novice to competent, but PBL graduates also described incidents at proficient level.

Chapter 9

A case-based curriculum

Leana R Uys

Introduction

Although case-based learning (CBL) is well known in business and law schools (Christensen et al., 1987), not much has been written about this as a curriculum development approach in nursing education. This is amazing, since it seems such an appropriate methodology for a clinical science.

In medical education, Cabot wrote a classic book about this approach in 1906, and there has been a consistent smattering of articles ever since (Glick and Amstrong, 1996; Schor et al., 1995). More recently there have also been a few references in dental education (Engel and Hendricks, 1994), and in the auxiliary health professions (van Leit, 1995).

The case-based learning curriculum model has been used in the preparation of nurse managers, as evidenced by the collection of such cases authored by Marquis and Huston (1994). In other nursing programmes, it is probably a method of teaching most educators use from time to time. A lecturer will illustrate a lecture by presenting a case study, or require students to reflect on their own practice by completing a case study. It is also sometimes used during clinical teaching. Some authors seem to use the term 'scenario' as an alternative to 'case'. For instance, the process described by Cascio et al. (1995) of enhancing critical skills in students by using practice-based scenarios seems to be identical with a case-based curriculum. The same term is also used by Manning et al. (1995), although they used the scenarios in a clinical role play simulation, and not for class discussion. The use of cases as the basis for a nursing curriculum needs further exploration.

Characteristics of case-based learning curricula

An integrated case-based curriculum

An integrated case-based curriculum is one in which students are given a set of complete cases for study and research in preparation for subsequent class discussions. All content components of the curriculum, that is, all subjects, may be integrated into the cases. The student's studying may be directed through study questions, and the finding of answers may be facilitated through identifying appropriate learning resources. The teacher facilitates the subsequent class discussion.

In a taxonomy of problem-based learning methods published in 1986, Barrows distinguishes between the case-based approach and similar approaches as follows:

Lecture-based case approach or case-based lecture approach

In a lecture-based case approach or case-based lecture approach, the content is presented through lectures, and one or two cases are used for illustration. The cases can be presented before or after the lecture, but it does not require self-study from students.

Case-based approach

In the case-based approach sequential management problems are used, in which students have to direct an inquiry and decide which informational and management options to follow. Although the level of inquiry may differ, this approach is similar to the problem-based approach, since both focus more strongly on the process of inquiry or learning.

Although cases may therefore be used in different ways in other types of curricula, the case-based curriculum is a specific type, which can be differentiated from others.

The characteristics of the case-based curriculum are therefore as follows:

- *It is a content-based curriculum:* It is a content-based curriculum, in the sense that the curriculum developers try to cover the required content through a series of integrated cases. There is, however, also a strong focus on the process of learning.
- *It is a self-directed curriculum:* It is a self-directed curriculum, in that students first confront the learning material by themselves. They study the problem and the new material and try to solve the problems before discussing them in class and validating their own thinking.
- *It structures knowledge in the clinical context:* It structures knowledge in the clinical context, which means that subsequent recall and use of the knowledge is facilitated (McKeachie, 1994). This aspect also acts as a motivator for learning, since adult learners are more interested in learning knowledge which is seen as relevant.
- *It is an integrated curriculum:* It is an integrated curriculum, in which a range of subjects can be presented around comprehensive cases. This allows students to see the relevance of biomedical and social sciences, and facilitates the application of knowledge in practice.

It is perhaps important to distinguish between a problem-based curriculum and case-based curriculum, since many of the authors writing on case development and use, link these two. Table 9.1 sets out the differences between these curriculum approaches.

Different authors have articulated the benefits of a case-based approach (Glendon and Ulrich, 1997; Jones, 1975; Levison et al., 1977; Rom and Mahler, 1986; Wynn, 1985):

1. It causes students to participate actively in the learning process.
2. It provides a real-life situation to which the student has to apply theoretical knowledge. This approach is in line with adult learning principles related to improved learning in situations where the knowledge is immediately applicable.
3. It demands decision-making and therefore forces students to make choices and explore the results of those choices. Students can practise difficult decision-making in conducive environments.
4. The analytical skills which students develop in this approach are increasingly demanded in nursing situations.
5. There are many opportunities in this approach for collaborative work in groups, which is also essential for contemporary health care.
6. There are few approaches to teaching/learning in which the socio-cultural aspects of health care can be so thoroughly integrated.
7. It allows for high student participation even with large classroom sizes. Discussion of the cases may take place in small groups or in large groups. In the classic application at Harvard Business School, classes of over 100 students often discuss the cases. This makes this approach more versatile and affordable than the problem-based approach.

Table 9.1 Comparison between a problem-based and a case-based curriculum

Concept	Problem-based curriculum	Case-based curriculum
Focus	Strongly on learning process	Balanced between content, process and outcomes
Information given	Limited information given. As students explore, additional information is released	Complete case information given before class session
Confronting the case	This is done in the group, students analysing the presenting problem together. Subsequent data collection and study are done individually	Students study the case individually first, before discussing it in class in a large group
Group size	Done in small groups, usually 8–12 students to one facilitator	May be done in large classes

8. It provides many opportunities for communication skills to be practised, including writing, presenting, debating, therapeutic and educational skills.
9. It involves students in reflecting on what they have done or decisions they have made.
10. Students respond favourably to this method.
11. The method is flexible, and can be adapted to suit different groups, subjects and situations.
12. Since the learning resources are identified for students, this curriculum can be used more easily than a problem-based curriculum in situations where students have difficulty accessing learning resources. This may be true in distance education and rural education.

Authors are not as forthcoming about the negative aspects of this approach. Dailey (1992) mentions the amount of time it takes to develop the cases as a major drawback, and Levison et al. (1977) also mentioned this. Argylis (1980) described a study of the actual process of case-based education, and identified dominance and control of sessions by facilitators, and facilitators protecting students and vice versa, instead of openly discussing problem issues. He then concludes that the method leads to conformity, error camouflage, risk mini-mization and face-saving. His criticism was subsequently strongly contested by Berger (1983) as based on flawed research design and reasoning. Wynn (1985) pointed out that cases were often over-simplified, so that they did not present reality, or were so complex that students could not handle them.

Case writing is hard work, time-consuming, requires intense study and demands emotional energy. It calls for competent facilitation skills from the facilitator and the students who have thoroughly studied the case and researched issues are prepared and eager to contribute in the case discussion. Without these ingredients, the use of cases can become superficial and the dis-cussion will lack in-depth criticism. Because patient data are usually complete in a CBL curriculum, as contrasted with PBL, this type of curriculum might not offer students adequate opportunity for developing inquiry skills.

Planning a case-based curriculum

The foundation of the curriculum process, during which the philosophy and theoretical framework are identified and the programme objectives described, remains the same. This phase still provides the foundation for the development of all subsequent stages, and gives direction to the development process. The next phase in the curriculum development process is the macro-curriculum stage, during which the curriculum is fleshed out and meaning and specificity are brought to the concepts and ideas. In this stage, the level objectives are developed, and then a content map is drawn for each level in the form of a case-study master plan. In the micro-curriculum development stage, the course plan-ning is done to put the curriculum concepts into practice. In the case-based curriculum educators have to decide on a case study protocol during this stage, and develop the different cases for study.

Case master plan

The content map is reflected in the case master plan, which lists the case content in broad outline. The objectives of the master plan are to:

- make sure that the major content is covered
- ensure that all subjects are integrated into each case
- ensure that the cases represent the client population adequately
- allow for sensitive sequencing of cases
- make sure that the curriculum strands are represented appropriately throughout the curriculum.

An example of a case master plan is provided in a brief article by Colby et al. (1986), in which the authors describe a course in social sciences and humanities which they developed for a medical programme. They used a case-based approach, and outlined the six cases they used in the form of a case study master plan. When developing a case master plan, the following steps are helpful:

1. Decide on content organizers, such as a theoretical framework or a nursing model, which will structure the courses. For instance, if a school decides to work on Orem's model, the first year nursing course cases can be built around self-care activities. This kind of organizing idea is essential to ensure coherence in the curriculum.
2. A decision is then made on the number of cases used in each level and course. If it is decided that a case should take about 1 month to work through, and there are 10 months in the academic year, ten cases can be planned. It is often practical to have cases of different magnitudes in the same course. Some outline does need to be decided upon.
3. At this stage it might be important to decide on the type of cases which will be included. If a course has the objective of introducing the student to the nursing process, using problem-solving triggers may be useful. If students are more junior, the kind of guidance to be given might be decided upon.
4. The last step in the development of the master plan is a brief outline of the content of each case, which should be enough to guide the case developers. The case descriptions should address issues such as patient demographics, healthcare setting, patient problems, nursing skills and any particular issue to be addressed in the case. Curricular strands, both vertical and horizontal are used to decide on case content.

Case protocol

The case studies on which the curriculum is based can vary greatly. In clinical nursing programmes it would probably be patients as cases, but each case could also include incidents which may reflect on administrative or educational issues around the client. In a management programme, a management situation would be sketched for analysis and study.

The case protocol is the pattern for each case, and it should not only follow a desired clinical reasoning pattern, but also fit with the conceptual framework on which the curriculum is based. Regan-Smith (1987: pp. 60–63) describes the use of cases in a medical curriculum, and outlines the assessment of the case presentations. The six assessment criteria actually represent what the faculty view as the essentials of a case, and are therefore similar to a case protocol. A case study protocol always consists of instructions to the student, case study (trigger) information (descriptions), student tasks (prescriptions) and learning resources.

Implementing a case-based learning curriculum

When using a case-based learning curriculum, students need to be prepared for using this methodology. They should be oriented to the principles of critical thinking, and the steps of the problem-solving process and decision-making. They have to be alerted to the need to incorporate previous knowledge and information from different scientific fields into the case. Another aspect that often needs reinforcement is that the student should not fall into generalizations, but should solve the specific problems of this case.

One also needs to build in mechanisms to ensure that students prepare the cases at home, and do not come into the class discussions hoping to pick up all the answers there. Students should be told what the expected preparation time for each case study is, and should be assisted to plan their professional and private lives to make time for this commitment. Such planning during the orientation period can make a significant difference later in the course. Once the course is under way, preparation can be encouraged by taking in a sample of case notes at the beginning of class, and making a copy for the teacher to mark. This can then count towards the student's final marks.

Principles underlying the implementation of case curriculum

The following are the principles underlying teaching by the case method (adapted from Cristensen and Hansen, 1987).

The primacy of situational analysis

The student studying via a case study is constantly confronted by the individual and the unique. In these situations, theory has to be applied, not just regurgitated, and the general has to be brought down to the specific. Christensen and Hansen (1987) refer to a sense for the critical, not only in analysing data, but also in prioritizing actions to be taken as essential to professional practice. In nursing this is particularly important, since the art of nursing has much to do with working with individuals and unique situations in a creative way. While the science of nursing underlies this practice, and brings to the situation the general laws, nursing goes beyond the general.

The imperative of relating analysis and action

While it is required of students to know, it is required of practitioners to act. The case study links these two. It leads the student to decide on action after analysis. This includes a willingness to make firm decisions on the basis of imperfect and limited data, and despite ever-present risk and uncertainty, to have the courage and self-confidence to carry out the proposed action (Christensen and Hansen, 1987).

Again, this applies directly to nursing. Even in situations which are relatively unclear, the practitioner often has to make a decision about what to do. Something has to be done, and doing nothing may have serious consequences.

The necessity of student involvement

'The active intellectual and emotional involvement of the student is the hallmark of case teaching' (Christensen and Hansen, 1987: p. 30). This involvement allows students to grow, and is inherently motivating.

Nursing is practice, and must be learnt by doing. This is not true only of psychomotor skills, but also of cognitive and inter-personal skills. The case method creates the opportunity to learn to read and understand, to observe, listen, diagnose, decide and contribute to group processes in achieving group goals.

A non-traditional instructor role

Instead of dispensing knowledge and demonstrating skill, the role of the group discussion facilitator is to guide the process of discovery in students. Although it might sometimes look as though the facilitator does very little, the active participation of the facilitator is essential.

Facilitators should ensure that the group reaches its goals, by keeping the proceedings orderly, and guiding discussion through skilled questioning. Preparation of facilitators for this new role is crucial for success. The method followed by the Harvard Medical School is an example of such an induction programme (Wetzel, 1996). They commence with a 2-hour orientation session, during which faculty is also given literature. This orientation is followed by practice tutorials for tutors, by experienced staff members. One week before the course begins, a course orientation meeting is held to discuss the course itself, course guides, assignments, cases and other material. The first case is also previewed. From then on, weekly meetings are held with new tutors to develop their skills further, and solve any problems they might have. Case previews and observation and feedback of sessions taken by the tutor are the mainstay of tutor development.

A balance of substantive and process teaching objectives

When applied successfully, the case method leads to students who have not only learnt adequate theory (content) on which to base their practice, but they have also learnt the process of their science. Each science has a perspective, a way of looking at data and using them. Students have to master this process as well as the information.

In nursing, the student should learn the process of analysing clinical situations from a nursing perspective. Nursing often uses the same theoretical base that other health sciences use, but in a unique way. This practice needs to be learnt.

The approach to the learning tasks promotes deep learning

It is now generally accepted that the way a student approaches a task determines whether deep or surface learning takes place (Cust, 1995). In the traditional lecture-based curriculum, the learning situation is structured so that the task seems to be 'listen to me and remember'. This leads to surface learning. In the case-based curriculum, the message seems to be 'read, think and solve the problems'. This leads to deep learning. Since the task is also presented in a holistic way, learning is holistic, and not atomistic.

Preparation for class interactions

A workbook which includes the course description, expected outcomes, course objectives, projects, assignments and their due dates, short notes on a case study approach, the case studies with questions or activities, reading material and evaluation tool for each class interaction should be made available to the students. The use of a case study approach should be discussed with the students, and the expectations and responsibilities of both the students and the facilitator clarified. This should be done about a week before the actual class interaction day. Learners need adequate time to go through the case and questions, to enhance class interaction. Giving the case to the students in advance is important because individuals read and grasp information at varying rates.

Each student is expected to give him or herself enough time to go over the case and tasks before coming to group discussions, to facilitate the efficient use of the instruction time. Class sessions are mainly for clarifying issues as well as sharing with the group the individual's interpretation of what was learned.

The students prepare for class as individuals. Individual preparation forces the student to think for him or herself, using their own opinions, experiences and resources to analyse the case and develop recommendations. The following guidelines should be given to the students to assist them in their preparation for class:

- Get a sense of the whole case first. Look at the title, the introduction, the headings, graphs, pictures, appendices, the central characters, what the story is about, case tasks or questions in the case, then read through the case. At the end, ask yourself what the case is really about and what is expected from you.
- Read the case again more carefully, bearing in mind the details you need to answer the study questions. While reading, mark the case, so that you will find the details later. Take notes to help you see the relationship in the information. Ask what additional information you need to work on the case tasks.
- Look at the questions again, find answers in the case and prepare literature to help you in justifying, explaining and presenting your responses.
- At the end, ask yourself what you have learned from the case and then prepare to present and defend your conclusions and present them convincingly.

Class activity in a case curriculum

Although the content of the curriculum is delivered via the case study, the classroom activities can be many and varied. Students prepare case material and come to class having studied the material, and practised the skills. The classroom can be used to achieve the following objectives.

1. Check whether students did the preparation, and if they did, whether they understood the material.
2. Give the students the opportunity to explore aspects of the material which they have not covered in the tasks.
3. Create an opportunity for experiential learning of skills.
4. Evaluate the level of performance achieved in tasks.

To achieve these objectives, there are different ways (detailed below) in which to structure classroom experiences.

Free discussion

In this class session, the students are invited to participate in a discussion without structuring it around the tasks they have had to perform. General questions may be asked to stimulate this kind of discussion, e.g. 'What did you think of this case? ', or 'What did you think about the situation the client was in?' or 'What do you think of the situation the nurse had to deal with?' This kind of open discussion can be effectively used to explore the attitudes, beliefs and fears of students.

Guided discussion

This discussion follows the tasks the student had prepared, with each task being discussed, problems ironed out, and final conclusions reached. This is useful when the material is very difficult, and it is essential to make sure that students master it.

Presentation and discussion

Instead of discussing the tasks in the open group, one student can be asked to present her/his task, and the discussion then follows the presentation. This allows students to learn to present material to a group, and also to defend their own work. Furthermore, it allows other students to learn how to criticize constructively, how to differ with a colleague, and how to argue on an issue.

The presentation need not be by an individual. The class can be divided into small groups, with each group discussing a different task. The small group explores the ways in which members complete the tasks, and each group has to reach consensus about the approach or answer. They then present their conclusion to the total class, and this is discussed. This allows for more participation from all members, and encourages students who find it difficult to participate in the large group. Cravener (1997: 21–26) describes how cases can be used as a teaching approach using small group discussions.

Demonstration

Demonstrations can be used in different ways in case-based curricula. The following are some examples:

- *Role play:* If students have prepared material which involves interpersonal skills, the class session can be used to ask students to display the skill by role playing. For instance, a teaching session can be demonstrated with one student playing the client, another the family members, and a third the nurse. Such role play sessions allow for formative evaluation, and also show students the level of preparation which is necessary in terms of skills development.

- *Product demonstration:* Student tasks sometimes involve making things, for instance a health education poster, or children's toy that stimulates a specific type of development in a toddler. During the classroom session such products can be displayed, discussed and evaluated. Class sessions can also be used to produce certain products, for instance, the group might be asked to produce a short play which can be used in health education. The class session is then used to plan, produce, discuss and evaluate the play.
- *Group role taking:* Group role taking is not really a role play exercise in as much as it is an experiential learning problem-solving exercise. When the case involves multiple clients and/or providers, the complexity of the situation and the skills necessary in dealing with it can be explored using this approach.

  The class group is divided into different small groups, each of which is allocated the 'role' of one of the clients or providers. They are given the task of preparing for a discussion with the other stakeholders by identifying what they want out of the meeting and why. When the groups of 'players' have planned their agendas the class is brought together for a 'meeting' during which each 'player/group' tries to achieve their objectives at the meeting. The group playing the nurse has to facilitate the meeting, while also trying to achieve the nursing objectives.

Self-study

Not all case-based curricula make use of class sessions in this manner. Morgan (1977) described a medical programme which was an independent studies programme and used complex case studies as one of its main teaching materials. Linke et al. (1977) also described a programme in which case studies were used as supplementary to the usual teaching approach, in this case the student worked the case, and then listened to a tape on which a faculty member discussed each task. This gave immediate feedback to enhance learning what is right, and not what is wrong.

Conclusion

The three central issues which determine the success or failure of the case-based approach to teaching/learning have been summarized as follows (Romm and Mahler, 1986):

1. the careful choice of interesting, thought-provoking cases by instructors
2. the in-depth preparation of the case by the instructor and students prior to discussion
3. flexibility and openness on the part of both facilitators and students during analysis of the case.

This approach to curriculum development can bring renewal to nursing education, but it is demanding in terms of preparation and implementation. With adequate time for preparation of cases and facilitators, and thorough planning for supported implementation, the three essentials could be achieved and more relevant and effective nursing education achieved.

Points for discussion

1. How should a first year and a last year case study differ? Why?
2. How much time should one allow for the preparation of the cases for one year of nursing studies?

References

Argyris, C. (1980) Some limitations of the case method: Experiences in a management development program. *Academy of Management Review*, 5(2): 291–298.

Barrows, H. S. (1986) A taxonomy of problem-based learning methods. *Medical Education*, 20: 481–486.

Berger, M. A. (1983) In defence of the case method: A reply to Argyris. *Academy of Management Review*, 8(2): 329–333.

Cascio, R. S., Campbell, D., Sandor, M. K., Rains, A. P. and Clark, M. C. (1995) Enhancing critical-thinking skills, faculty–student partnerships in community health nursing. *Nurse Educator*, 20(2), 38–43.

Christensen, C. R. and Hansen, A. J. (1987) *Teaching and the Case Method*. Boston, MA: Harvard Business School.

Colby, K. K., Thomas, P., Almy, M. D. and Aubkoff, M. (1986) Problem-based learning of social sciences and humanities by fourth-year medical students. *Journal of Medical Education*, 61: 413–415.

Cravener, P. A. (1997). Promoting active learning in large lecture classes. *Nurse Educator* 22(3): 21–26.

Cust, J. (1995) A relational view of learning: implications for nurse education. *Nurse Education Today*, 16(4): 256–266.

Dailey, M. A. (1992). Developing case studies. *Nurse Educator*, 17(3): 8–11.

Engel, F. E. and Hendricson, W. D. (1994) A case-based model in orthodontics. *Journal of Dental Education*, 58(10): 762–767.

Glendon, K. and Ulrich, D. L. (1997) Unfolding cases and experiential learning model. *Nurse Educator*, 22(4): 15–18.

Glick, T. H. and Amstrong, E. G. (1996) Crafting cases for problem-based learning: experience in a neuroscience course. *Medical Education*, 30(1): 24–30.

Jones, R. F. (1975) The case study method. *Journal of Chemical Education*, 52(7): 460–461.

Levison, D. A., Fawkes, J. B., MacGillivray, S. and Beck, J. (1977) Problem solving cases in teaching of applied pathology. *Medical Education*, 11: 21–24.

Linke, A. A., Irwin, M. D., Frank, M. D., Abraham, T. K., Cockett, M. D. and Vernon Netto, I. C. (1977) Case studies for medical students. *Journal of Medical Education*, 48: 584.

Manning, J., Broughton, V. and McConnell, E. A. (1995) Reality based scenarios facilitate knowledge network development. *Contemporary Nurse*, 4(1): 16–21.

Marquis, B. L. and Huston, C. J. (1994) *Management Decision Making for Nurses*, 2nd edn. Philadelphia, PA: J. B. Lippincott Co.

McKeachie W. J. (1994) *Teaching Tips*, 9th edn. Lexington, D.C. Heath and Co.

Morgan, H. R. (1977) A problem-oriented independent studies programme in basic medical sciences. *Medical Education*, 11: 394–398.

Regan-Smith, M. D. (1987) Teaching clinical reasoning in a clinical clerkship by use of case assessments. *Journal of Medical Education*, 62: 60–63.

Romm, T. and Mahler, S. (1986) A three dimensional model for using case studies in the academic classroom. *Higher Education*, 15: 677–696.

Schor, N. F., Troen, P., Adler, S., Williams, J. G., Knater, S. L. and Mahling, D. E. (1995) Integrated case studies and medical decision making – a novel, computer-assisted bridge from the basic sciences to the clinics. *Academic Medicine,* 70(9): 814–817.

van Leit, B. (1995) Using the case method to develop clinical reasoning skills in problem-based learning. *American Journal of Occupational Therapy* 49(4): 349–353.

Wetzel, M. S. (1996) Developing the role of the tutor/facilitator. *Postgraduate Medical Journal*, 72: 474–477.

Wynn, M. (1985) *Planning Games – Case Study Simulations in Land Management and Development*. New York: E. & F.N. Spon.

Recommended reading

Cravener, P. A. (1997) Promoting active learning in large lecture classes. *Nurse Educator*, 22(3): 21–26.

Although the author does not deal with case-based curriculum, she illustrates how one can use a case teaching approach with large groups of students.

Glendon, K. and Ulrich, D. L. (1997) Unfolding cases: and experiential learning model. *Nurse Educator*, 22(4): 15–18.

This article gives useful examples of cases, and a checklist for use during case construction.

Dailey, M. A. (1992) Developing case studies. *Nurse Educator*, 17(3): 8–11.

This is a short article which also gives useful steps in the process of case development.

Chapter 10

Developing problem scenarios and cases

Marilyn B Lee and Leana R Uys

Introduction

When developing a problem-based learning (PBL) curriculum, the micro-curriculum consists to a large extent of problem scenarios. When developing a case-based curriculum (CBC), the micro-curriculum consists to a large extent of case scenarios. Although these two micro-curriculum components are similar, there are differences in the methods of development of scenarios. Together with facilitator preparation and characteristics (Haith-Cooper, 2003; Leung and Lee, 2003), the quality of the scenario used to focus student learning is an important consideration in problem- or case-based teaching strategies. A systematic, competent approach to the development of scenarios is one of the keys to enhancing the quality and efficacy of these teaching strategies (Glew, 2003; Washington *et al.*, 2003). In this chapter strategies for development of both micro-curriculum components are described.

Components of an effective problem scenario

It is generally accepted that problem scenarios are comprised of:

- a scenario or vignette
- reference file of resources
- facilitator guide.

A detailed description of each of these components is provided in this section.

The scenario or vignette

The scenario presents a brief description of a clinical or practical case that is relevant to the learner. The scenario provides a description of a situation on which the learner can focus, generate hypotheses, identify areas of knowledge gap and develop realistic, achievable learning objectives. Information provided in the scenario is sufficient to stimulate the learner but is not exhaustive.

Moreover, intentional gaps in information are part of the problem scenario. Constructing the scenario with gaps in information stimulates learners to recognize what knowledge they have that is relevant to the problem situation and promotes identification of learning needs. Identification of learning needs creates motivation to explore additional concepts thus fostering learner engagement, a sense of personal responsibility for learning, as well as development of life-long learning skills (Smith, 2002). In addition, this technique is effective in creating continuous motivation for new knowledge development.

It may be helpful to the teaching staff writing problem scenarios to view the technique of leaving gaps in information as a 'phased-in' approach, keeping in mind that additional information will be provided at a later time. 'Phased in' refers to a technique in which information is revealed as the learner discovers that the information is required. For example, the learner may be given a problem scenario where the client is seen in the clinic with complaints of excessive thirst, polyuria and fatigue. The learner is expected to identify hypotheses that could realistically explain these complaints. In order to determine which of the hypotheses is most likely, the learner identifies knowledge gaps and develops learning objectives. In the process of achieving learning objectives the learner realizes that blood chemistry values are needed. At this point the learner requests this information from the facilitator. The information, available in the scenario facilitator guide, is provided to the learner at that time as the second 'phase' of the problem scenario. This technique continues throughout the problem scenario until the learner has requested and received all the necessary and available information from the facilitator. In this manner the facilitator is able to ensure that the learner deals with the essential concepts at a level appropriate to his/her learning.

Three essential elements in the process of development of problem scenarios are validation, modification and updating. These elements should be performed on a continuous basis to ensure that scenarios stimulate learning of the essential content and enable learners to meet course objectives. Validation, ensuring that the scenario addresses essential concepts, can be achieved by involving content experts in scenario development and testing (Amos and White, 1998). Another method that is useful in ensuring valid and effective problem scenarios is using chart data combined with clinical experience in the development of problem scenarios.

Modification should occur when evaluators determine that the scenario needs alteration and should focus on the areas suggested by the evaluator. Teaching staff may also determine that modification is necessary if the scenario does not elicit the intended motivation for learning of specific concepts. Finally, updating must occur on a regular basis because new knowledge is continually being generated. It is expected that problem-based learning will motivate and enable students to access new information and the scenarios should guide learners in identifying this new knowledge as a gap in their own knowledge (Grabinger and Dunlap, 2002).

Reference file of resources

The development of a reference file is also an essential element in problem-based scenario development. Both learners and facilitators use this file. The file should include all available resources, including literature (books, journals and online information), professionals, community members, etc., and relevant organizations (Edwards et al., 1998). Because the efficient use of the problem solving process is expected to enable learners to create and acquire knowledge, the resource file must support this endeavour.

There are four advantages to the development and use of a resource file, it: (a) widens student selection of resources, (b) enhances learners' understanding of the contextual nature of knowledge, (c) highlights areas of knowledge gap and (d) promotes the use of a wider selection of resources in future problem solving tasks. Learners, especially those in the early years of study, often do not consider the variety of resources available to them and the advantage that using them can bring, thus they tend to utilize a very narrow selection of resources, especially written resources. The information in the resource file highlights to the student the other options available to them to gain information in order to construct new knowledge. Using a variety of resources also enhances the learner's understanding of the contextual dimensions of a concept. This outcome occurs because the learner obtains a variety of perspectives on a problem, thus reinforcing the importance of context and promoting storage and retrieval for future problem-solving tasks, especially in similar contexts. A third advantage in obtaining a variety of perspectives related to a concept is that the resources often highlight to the learners areas of further gaps in knowledge, thus motivating the learners to explore the concepts in greater depth. In theory, the more varied the resources used by learners the greater the breadth and depth of knowledge acquired in relation to the essential concept. Finally, learners who are accustomed to using a wide variety of resources are more likely to be able to apply these habits to future problems in practice. Examples of the kind of resources that would appear in a resource file for a problem scenario on diabetes mellitus would include recent literature on etiology and treatments, diabetologists or endocrinologists in the community, nursing personnel working with diabetic patients, community support groups and diabetic teaching information.

Facilitator's guide

The primary rationale for the recommended components in problem-based learning scenarios is to provide adequate support to students and facilitators. One advantage in having the facilitator guide is that, when developed satisfactorily, facilitators do not have to be experts in the clinical area of the problem scenario (Matthes et al, 2002; Ravens et al, 2002). There is considerable debate regarding expert versus non-expert facilitators, however, in one author's experience, if adequate facilitator guides are provided a generalist can utilize the guide to guide the student's learning competency. Moreover, if the facilitator is willing and able to acknowledge his/her own knowledge gaps, learners can gain from observing the facilitator's problem-solving strategies.

The facilitator's guide should contain at a minimum:

- essential concepts to be addressed by the learner (Correa et al, 2003)
- likely and possible responses of a student at different points in the problem solving process (Cooke and Donovan, 1998)
- background and resource information that may be needed by the facilitator.

Essential concepts to be addressed by the learners

This component of the facilitator's guide includes a list of concepts that are to be addressed by the student in the problem-solving exercise. The list can be broken into essential and relevant concepts. Prioritizing concepts in this manner assists the facilitator to ensure that at least the essential concepts are addressed in the learning experience. The list of priorities also highlights to the facilitators areas in which they may have knowledge deficits and may need to determine their own learning objectives. Using the previous example of a client with diabetes mellitus, the essential concepts of glucose metabolism, immune function, heredity/genetics in disease, circulation, neurological function, sterile technique and assessment of learning readiness could be essential concepts in the facilitators' guide. Other concepts that may be identified could include growth and development and the economic and psychosocial impact of chronic illness. These concepts might also change in priority depending on the type of programme, or qualifications of the student, or the student's level in the programme.

Likely and possible responses of students at different points in the problem-solving process

Identification of likely and possible responses of students helps to prepare the facilitator for the guidance role. Students' responses are an indicator of what and how they are thinking. If the responses are not listed or if a student does not address issues as predicted, this omission *may* indicate that there are serious flaws in the student's thinking or *may* indicate knowledge gaps not identified previously by the learner. The facilitator, however, must be open to other ways of viewing a problem. It must also be recognized that in spite of validation and testing, other responses may be appropriate but missing from the facilitator's guide.

Responses that would be likely from a learner viewing the diabetes mellitus scenario described previously could include:

1. 'These must be signs and symptoms of some disorder.' (Hypothesis)
2. 'Does anyone know what these symptoms could be caused by?' (Exploring knowledge gaps)
3. 'Where can we go to get this information? Why don't you and Amanda go to the library and look in the medical dictionary. Mary and I will go to see the nurse in the medical clinic.' (Setting learning objectives).

Finally, included in this section of the facilitator guide may be suggested questions that the facilitator could pose in order to promote greater depth and breadth in the learner's thinking.

Background and resource information that may be needed by the facilitator

In cases where the problem scenario requires specialized knowledge, non-expert facilitators will require background knowledge and resource information (Maudsley, 2003). This component of the problem scenario is essential to ensuring that the facilitator is able to guide the learner to benefit optimally from the process.

Guidelines for development of problem scenarios

Given that the problem scenarios are expected to drive students' learning, the following guidelines are suggested in order to develop problem scenarios that enhance achievement of expected learning. In most cases the rationale for the guidelines is based on one or all of the philosophical underpinnings. The guidelines are as follows.

- the design of the problem should be intentional
- the problem should be realistic
- adequate information should be provided
- a facilitator guide should be developed.

Problem design is intentional

The problem scenario should reflect the aims and terminal objectives of the curriculum and lead the student to opportunities for learning essential concepts for a practitioner at the level at which the learner is studying. In addition, the problem scenario, over the length of the programme, should enable the learner to master the skills required of a graduate of the programme. If the curriculum clearly delineates the essential concepts and skills in each course, the scenario can be designed to motivate learners to master these concepts and skills. For example, most nursing curricula include pathophysiology of the endocrine system in essential concepts, specifically, the pathophysiology of diabetes mellitus. In addition, the ability to assess, make nursing diagnoses, formulate plans, implement nursing interventions (such as giving a subcutaneous injection) and evaluate patient progress related to the problem is expected. Beyond these concepts are psychosocial and biological concepts such as coping, self-care, hereditary aspects of disease and developmental considerations. These concepts can all be integrated into the problem scenario by selecting an actual case that includes these issues.

Realistic problem situation

The problem scenario should reflect a problem or issue that could actually arise in professional practice. One significant reason for creating realistic problem scenarios is that this strategy has the potential to facilitate a learner to move from understanding abstract concepts to application of these concepts in practice, in other words, bridge the theory–practice gap. Another reason for developing realistic problem scenarios is the increased facility with which a learner can retrieve information in future clinical problem situations. Finally, student engagement and motivation to learn is significantly increased with the degree of realism present in the problem (Grabinger and Dunlap, 2002; Khoo, 2003). Many programmes that use problem-based learning enhance the realism of the problem scenarios by developing simulations. McMaster University in Canada, the forerunner in PBL for nursing and medical education, utilizes the theatre arts of other students as well as local amateur performers to create realistic problem simulations. Use of simulations is especially effective because students have an opportunity to practise clinical skills such as interviewing and counselling, as well as test hypotheses, with 'clients' throughout the problem-solving process.

Use of actual patient case data, while ensuring confidentiality, is also an effective strategy for the development of realistic problem scenarios. When the essential concepts are identified, scenario developers can collaborate with clinical experts to identify existing or past clinical cases that can guide the learner to acquire knowledge of the essential concepts. It is useful sometimes to have several health disciplines represented in the group that is developing scenarios for courses. In most cases, an actual clinical situation can be identified, data obtained and a realistic scenario developed from the data.

Adequate information

Supporting information is essential to ensuring that there is not premature closure of the problem (Cooke and Donovan, 1998). This information can often be given in the form of additional data that the student is expected to request (the 'phased in' approach) as they identify gaps in their knowledge. Problem scenarios should have 'triggers' imbedded in the scenario that increase a student's use of previous knowledge and stimulate critical thinking. For example, polyuria should trigger use of knowledge of osmosis and osmolality from the students' biochemistry course.

If learners do not recognize that there is a gap in their knowledge or if the level of information obtained is inadequate, the facilitator must perform a quality assurance role. The facilitator must confront inadequate or incorrect information. Development of problem-solving skills depends on the quality and quantity of information contained in the scenario, a student's inquiry skills and the manner in which a learner is guided in obtaining information (Haith-Cooper, 2003; Johnston and Tinning, 2001).

Components of an effective case

A case always consists of the following components:

1. guidelines for the student
2. case (trigger) information (description)
3. student tasks (prescription)
4. learning resources.

A detailed description of each of these components is provided in this section.

Guidelines for the student

This section acts as an advanced organizer to assist the student with the task at hand. In an unguided case, the instructions might be quite limited, e.g., 'Study this case in the light of the unit objectives'. In a guided case instructions can be in the form of objectives, or general instructions. It is important that it is made clear to the students what they should do before class, and what will be done in class. If this is not done carefully, students may not prepare adequately, expecting to work through the case in class. Guided instructions could be 'Study each description and complete the tasks as set out. Please complete all readings, and do not just read until you have the solution to the case problem. Remember that you will have to deal with other clients with different problems in future.'

Case or trigger information (description)

This component is usually given in a progressive way, so that only relevant information is given before the appropriate action is elicited from the student; much like the 'phased-in' approach described for problem-based learning scenario development. Furthermore, it is important to make the case study material as close to real life as possible, without making it too complex for beginning practitioners to deal with.

Student tasks (prescription)

After each set of case study materials, the student is required to answer specific questions, prepare material, analyse material or research a topic. The following tasks are examples:

- prepare an induction programme for new staff on the unit
- criticize a specific policy document
- prepare a lesson plan to teach this patient . . .
- write out your own thinking on this ethical dilemma in the following format . . . .

Learning resources

Students are referred to specific learning resources. Depending on how accessible these are, students may be required to identify and find resources independently, or they may be supplied. The more advanced students' learning skills become, the more extensive the requirements might be, or the more limited the references may become.

As with the problem-based scenario, another element which might be included in every case study is a facilitator's guide. This component contains information prepared to assist the facilitator in dealing with the case study. The facilitator's guide may include information about the 'solutions' to the case study, tips about how to use classroom sessions and additional information about the issues raised in the case.

Guidelines for the development of cases

In a traditional content-based curriculum, the delivery of lectures is the central element which determines the quality of the teaching. In a case-based curriculum, the essential element determining quality is the case. Development of a good case is a task which demands time and attention. The following steps should be taken in the development of cases.

Planning

The first step in the planning is to establish tentative hypotheses about what could be included in the case, and how the case could be structured, based on the case description in the case master plan (see Chapter 9). For instance, if the case is about a 45-year-old man who has a spinal injury, the tentative hypotheses might be anxiety due to potential paralysis as well as the pathophysiology of this kind of injury. Both concepts are important issues for students to study. Furthermore, one could hypothesize that reaction to injury and nursing care of a person who is bedridden might be usefully covered in this case. Other issues that might be important to address include: problems with elimination, and family reactions and involvement. The list of tentative hypotheses assists the case developers to target their interviewing and chart reviews, so that data for the case are more comprehensive and realistic.

Given the type of client the case is about, and the tentative hypotheses, the developers plan where they will find information on which to build the case. The potential sources include clients with these clinical conditions, their families and caregivers, client records, the literature and service statistics. Decisions are made about how many people to interview, and whether they should be hospital-based or community-based or both. It cannot be over-emphasized that cases must be based on real data collected for the purpose of developing a specific case. Attention to this requirement is the only way in which cases have a reality and immediacy that engages the student. Developers should resist the temptation to sit in their offices and make up cases based on vaguely remembered experiences from the past.

Collect case data

Most cases are developed from a number of real cases put together. For instance, from one client the developer might use the family situation and home care problems, while using the clinical data of another client. Together these data make an interesting case, while individually each leaves out concepts that are essential for the student to study.

Real case material is used to enliven the case study. When the developer is building a case file, pictures of the patient, wounds, family home, and other important aspects of the case can be included. Laboratory reports, ECG and X-rays are further material which might be included in the case. In addition, sometimes an interview with a consenting client or family member might be video- or audio-taped and used as a learning activity. It is also important to have samples of nursing care items available for students to look at and inspect. For instance, incontinence aids should be available for viewing for a case study dealing with incontinence.

It is important to collect data widely enough to illustrate not only an individual's problems, but also the wider context of those problems. For instance, the reactions, attitudes and situations of family members may play a crucial role in the care and cure of the client, and should not be neglected when developing a case. Often the same is true about healthcare professionals, i.e., they sometimes have attitudes and problems which influence their care of clients, and such information should also be included in cases. An example of attitudinal influence on healthcare professionals is the problem which staff of trauma units have about caring for people after suicide attempts. Acknowledging this attitudinal problem may not be enough, and more information on the problem might need to be explored. Furthermore, in some cases it is important for students to get an idea of how common a problem is, and therefore additional data, such as morbidity figures, might have to be collected. Finally, the general attitude of society might influence care, and this needs to be researched in the literature to form part of the case. An example of how individual and societal attitudes influences care is the current debate about the care of clients with HIV/AIDS in southern Africa.

Finalize the case

Once the case data have been collected, the case is 'put together'. The final decisions about what to include, and what to eliminate, are made. The case description is then prepared, and the student tasks formulated.

Although these activities sound straightforward, it can be quite difficult to organize the data rationally and still maintain the comprehensiveness of the case. One approach that could be useful is to chart the nursing decisions which will have to be made in the case in the form of a decision chart that answers questions, e.g., 'What is the priority problem?', 'What should be done about this problem?', 'What then?'. This kind of chart could be used to structure the case (Bieron and Frank, 1998).

It is important that there be some flexibility in the final development of the case. Developers often come across very rich data during data collection, and it is a pity if such data are lost because the developers remain strictly to the case master plan. For instance, if the developers interview a client about mobility problems, and are given very interesting data on incontinence, it might be possible to incorporate this problem into the case rather than adhere strictly to the original plan. A holistic approach is important in case development, and making cases holistic enriches learning. Moreover, if students meet the same problem in different forms, contexts or in different clients, they may be better prepared.

The format in which a case is presented can differ widely. For example, one group used a display which included posters, microscopes with slides, X-rays and photographs and specimens. This approach was used to teach applied pathology (Linke et al., 1973). Many cases are presented to students in the form of duplicated handouts. However, these can be augmented by other material which is centrally displayed or available, such as video- or audio-cassettes, pictures, objects, etc. Indeed, tutors can even place information on a web page for students to access at any time.

It is usually when the case is in the final stages that decisions about the case identifiers are made. A case identifier is the system used by a school to identify cases, e.g., each case will have the following case data as case identifiers:

- course home: e.g., fundamental nursing
- case number e.g., case 3
- case focus: e.g., elimination and psychosocial needs
- case title: e.g., Mr Perge.

Review the case against established criteria

It is useful for the faculty to develop a case evaluation checklist which identifies the main criteria to which all cases should adhere. These criteria will differ widely according to the type of programme and the conceptual framework decided upon by the faculty. For instance, one school had the following criteria. Every scenario should include:

- a family genogram
- pictures and other information aimed at making the case 'real'
- cultural and life-span details
- focus not only on the individual care, but also on group/aggregate issues, such as health policy
- information to assist the student to identify all role-players, both in terms of the client group and the provider group.

Such a list of criteria is extremely important, since it ensures that curriculum strands are consistently present. The list can focus on both content and process of an educational programme, and therefore ensures a balanced approach in the teaching.

Another important task when reviewing a case is to make use of subject specialists, level specialists, health service providers and students. Consulting librarians and checking the resource list would also be useful when performing the final check.

Conclusion

Problem- and case-based learning are effective processes used in the education of nurses in a number of institutions around the globe. The effectiveness of these learning processes is dependent on the quality of the problem or case scenarios used to facilitate learning. The skill of developing effective problem scenarios or case studies is therefore as important for nurse educators to master as the more traditional lecturing or demonstrating.

Points for discussion

1. How and why would different types of curricula be combined to deliver a nursing programme?
2. What essential resources are needed in the library to support a BPL or a CBL curriculum?

References

Amos, E. and White, M. J. (1998) Teaching tools: problem-based learning. *Nurse Educator*, 23(2): 11–14, 21.

Bieron, J. F. and Frank, J. D. (1998) *Case Studies Across a Science Curriculum*. Online. Available at: http://ublib. Buffalo.edu/libraries/projects/cases/curriculum.html.

Cooke, M. and Donovan, A. (1998) The nature of the problem: the intentional design of problems to facilitate different levels of student learning. *Nurse Education Today*, 19: 462–469.

Correa, B. B., Pinto, P. R. and Rendas, A. B. (2003) How do learning issues relate with content in a problem-based learning pathophysiology course? *Advances in Physiology Education*, 27(2): 62–69.

Edwards, N. C., Hebert, D., Moyer, A., Peterson, J., Sims-Jones, N. and Verhovsek, H. (1998) Problem-based learning: preparing post-RN students for community-based care. *Journal of Nursing Education*, 37(3): 139–141.

Glew, R. H. (2003) The problem with problem-based medical education. Promises not kept. *Biochemistry and Molecular Biology Education*, 31(1): 52–56.

Grabinger, S. and Dunlap, J. C. (2002) Problem-based learning as an example of active learning and student engagement. Advances in information systems. *Lecture Notes in Computer Science*, 2457: 375–384.

Haith-Cooper, M. (2003) An exploration of tutor's experiences of facilitating problem-based learning. Part 2 – Implications for the facilitation of problem-based learning. *Nurse Education Today*, 23(1): 65–75.

Johnston, A. K. and Tinning, R. (2001) Meeting the challenge of problem-based learning: developing the facilitators. *Nurse Education Today*, 21: 161–169.

Khoo, H. E. (2003) Implementation of problem-based learning in Asian medical schools and students' perceptions of their experience. *Medical Education*, 37(5): 401–409.

Leung, K. K. and Lee, M. B. (2003) Development of a teaching style inventory for tutor evaluation in problem-based learning. *Medical Education*, 37(5): 410–416.

Linke, C. A., Frank, I., Cockett, A. T. K. and Netto, I. C. V. (1973) Case studies for medical students. *Journal of Medical Education*, 48(6): 584.

Matthes, J., Marxen, B., Linke, R. M., Antepohl, W., Coburger, S., Christ, H., Lehmacher, W. and Herzig, S. (2002) The influence of tutor qualification on the process and outcome of learning in a problem-based course of basic medical pharmacology. *Archives of Pharmacology*, 366: 58–63.

Maudsley, G. (2003) The limits of tutors' comfort zones with four integrated knowledge themes in a problem-based undergraduate medical curriculum (interview study). *Medical Education*, 37(5): 417–423.

Ravens, U., Nitsche, I., Haag, C. and Dobrev, D. (2002) What is a good tutorial from a student's point of view? Evaluation of tutorials in a newly established PBL block course 'Basics of Drug Therapy'. *Archives of Pharmacology*, 366: 69–76.

Smith, H. C. (2002) A course director's perspective on problem-based learning curricula in biochemistry. *Academic Medicine*, 77(12): 1189–1198.

Washington, E. T., Tysubger, J. W., Snell, L. M. and Palmer, L. R. (2003) Developing and evaluating ambulatory care: problem-based learning cases. *Medical Teacher*, 25(2): 136–141.

Recommended reading

Gwele, N. S., Uys, L. R. and Majumdar, B. (2001) An analysis of facilitator contributions in PBL groups. *International Nursing Perspectives*, 1(2–3): 94–104.
This article reports on a qualitative research project analyzing the quantity and quality of facilitator interventions in PBL groups, and the effect on the functioning of the groups.

Chapter 11

Developing a community-based nursing education curriculum

Ntombifikile G Mtshali

Introduction

The role of health professionals throughout the world is undergoing significant changes due to the reorientation of healthcare systems towards the World Health Organization's (WHO) goal of 'Health for All' through primary health-care (PHC). When considering the development of the health professional, the WHO (1985) asserted that health personnel were not appropriately trained for the tasks they were expected to perform in society, and that the planning of their education remained isolated from consumer needs and the needs of the health-care service (WHO, 1993). Health professionals in hospital-based education have minimal preparation in the wider aspects of health, and they have little opportunity to learn how to address the social, economic and political forces affecting health. In the words of McWhinney 'A student whose sole experience of illness has been in hospital, has seen a small fraction of the illness of the people, and in hospital the patient is isolated from the context of his or her ill-ness, namely the family and social dimensions of the ill health' (1980: p. 189). The conventional method of training students in hospitals is thus no longer regarded as an appropriate method of developing graduates, who should be responsive to the needs of the society as a whole. Several innovative teaching approaches to the education of health professionals have been proposed. Community-based education (CBE) seems one promising approach to enhance the relevance of education to the needs of the population, as CBE is founded on a PHC philosophy.

Conceptualization of community-based education

Literature suggests that there is no consensus on what the concept CBE means, as this term is defined differently by a number of authors and sometimes is used interchangeably with a number of other terms, such as community-oriented education, population-based education, or service learning. In this chapter, the WHO's (1987) definition will be used. Community-based education is viewed as a means of achieving educational relevance to community needs and, consequently, as a way of implementing a community-oriented educational programme. CBE consists of learning activities that utilize the community extensively as a learning environment, in which not only the students, but also the teachers, members of the community, and representatives of other sectors are actively involved throughout the educational experience. The WHO further maintains that, depending on how the population is distributed, CBE can be conducted wherever people live, in a rural, suburban, or urban area, and wherever it can be organized. According to the WHO, an educational programme can be called community-based if, for the entire duration of the programme, it includes an appropriate number of learning activities in a balanced variety of settings, namely, in the community and in a diversity of healthcare services at all levels, including tertiary care hospitals. The distribution of community-based learning activities throughout the duration of the curriculum is an essential characteristic of a community-based education programme (WHO, 1987: p. 9).

Core characteristics of CBE

CBE programmes exhibit a number of characteristics of which some are regarded as core characteristics distinguishing CBE programme from hospital-based programmes. These discriminating characteristics include but are not limited to those outlined below.

The primacy of community as a learning environment

The community as a clinical learning environment is used to the extent that the percentage of community-based learning experiences outweighs learning experiences in other clinical learning settings. Ideally, community-based learning activities should be 50% or more of the whole programme, with the students repeatedly exposed to community-based learning experiences to facilitate the development of competencies and interest in serving in such settings. In CBE the community is regarded as more than just a learning space, because of its contribution to the preparation of graduates. This setting exposes students to live dynamic contexts, conscientizing them to the socio-economic, political, cultural and other factors influencing the health of individuals, families and the community. Such exposure is believed to facilitate a better understanding of social issues and it equips students with the skills required to deal with such community issues or problems. More importantly, it provides a complete or comprehensive holistic view of health and illness, which is missed out when patients are encountered in hospital settings only.

Timing of first community exposure

CBE requires early exposure of students to community-based learning experiences, so as to familiarize them with community settings first (not just any community settings but under-served communities) where PHC is the main focus of practice. The students are introduced to these settings first before being placed in tertiary healthcare settings, in order to understand healthy individuals in their natural settings and how their surroundings impact on their health. Furthermore, it is believed that the students should be socialized to PHC as early as possible, to change their mindset about primary health care which has been viewed to be less important than curative care. Although early exposure to community-based learning experiences might be viewed as 'early indoctrination' of students into PHC, early exposure to community-based learning experiences is believed to facilitate the building of a good and solid PHC foundation. The culture of health promotion and illness prevention is then developed as early as possible in the students.

Sequencing of learning experiences

Learning experiences in CBE are vertically organized, from healthy individuals in their natural settings (families and communities), to PHC clinics where health promotion and illness prevention are the area of focus, to hospitalized sick clients in tertiary healthcare settings. Such sequencing of learning experiences allows for the development of competencies required at each level of health care, ensuring that the students build on previous experiences in their increasingly complex learning experiences, accumulating experience required at each level of health care. Such sequencing of learning experiences also promotes understanding of different levels of health care and their functioning relationship. The learning experiences in a curriculum might be organized in the following manner:

- first year: community settings (home visits, family studies, community assessment and health promotion and illness prevention activities)
- second year: comprehensive or primary healthcare clinics (entry level to hospital, health promotion and illness prevention activities, attending to minor ailments, referral, etc.)
- third year: hospital-based learning (general nursing, curative focus and some rehabilitation)
- fourth year: year of specialization (midwifery and mental health nursing units).

Service provision

CBE encourages learning through providing service to the community. The service provided should address the priority health needs of the community. Hence, CBE is viewed as one way of making health care accessible to those communities with limited health resources. Engaging in such learning experiences promotes learning that is meaningful in that students develop a better understanding of what is expected in their future careers. It is during the process of service delivery that students develop work-related competencies by engaging in learning experiences which closely resemble those activities of professionals in real-life settings. The service provided should however have a clear educational focus, as learning is the main purpose of providing service. Quinn et al. (2000) emphasized that academic institutions have an ethical obligation to see to the interests of the students, therefore providing service should be secondary to learning.

Community involvement

The success of CBE depends on the community's willingness and readiness to participate in the preparation of students. A community-oriented curriculum requires the use of problems drawn from the community to form part of the curriculum content. The community can help students identify the health problems in the community and learn more about them. Both the community and students should benefit from community-based learning. Ezzat (1995) outlined some principles which should be considered when working with communities.

These principles include:

- Community members have the right to share the responsibility of community based learning activities; their contribution is central, both to the learning phase and to the implementation of action programmes.
- Students cannot use communities as if they were laboratories (spaces which one can use as an object), and students should therefore accept their responsibility towards the community.
- Partnership, rather than paternalism, should dominate the interaction process between academic institutions and communities.
- The role of the community in students' learning has to be accurately defined and planned according to established goals and objectives.
- The students–community links should start early in the educational experience and must continue throughout (Ezzat, 1995: p. 134)
- Community-based programmes must be of clear benefit to both the students and the community in which they are implemented. This implies effective community contribution to the educational programme.

Collaboration between the healthcare system and the academic institution

Community-based education is characterized by an academic institution that works closely with the healthcare system. This collaboration should begin as early as the time of conducting the situational analysis. Collaboration between the healthcare system (not just the hospital) and academic institution is one way to address the priority healthcare needs of the community and to enhance relevance of education to the needs of the healthcare system (WHO, 1993). This collaboration bridges the gap between the academic institution and the health-care system and the gap between the required consumer needs and expectations. As a warning, Al Refai (1995) highlighted some possible problems that might be a threat to a collaborative effort, such as:

- differences in objectives and responsibilities of these two institutions
- financial implications of the collaboration
- lack of political interest and support for the initiative
- traditionalism that centres health professionals' education and health care providers
- a public that does not easily accept changes in the traditional pattern of service.

Other problems may result from limited knowledge about the benefits of collaboration and the contribution of each partner to the collaboration; and power struggle between these two parties, with the health service sector anxious about being dominated by the academic institution. Efforts should be made to deal with these problems as early as possible.

Multidisciplinary team approach

CBE is aimed at producing professionals who will be able to function in inter-disciplinary teams, and exposing students to multidisciplinary team learning facilitates this. The students learn to understand their roles within a team and the functions of other team members. Using a multidisciplinary approach allows for the sharing of expertise to the best advantage, increases communication among teachers, learners from different disciplines and from the health service staff, and permits collective assessment, allocation and utilization of educational resources according to needs (WHO, 1987). Through functioning in teams the students develop professionally, as this necessitates respect, trust and commitment from team members.

Problem-centred learning

Problem-centred learning is viewed as a vehicle for enabling students to develop usable bodies of integrated knowledge and problem-solving skills. The students learn to deal with real-life problems which are work-related. In CBE health problems prevalent in clinical settings form the basis for learning and teaching and these problems interconnect strongly with the content covered in class. Other important characteristics in CBE include intersectoral linkages where students learn to function in intersectoral teams especially when addressing community problems. Valid performance assessment is assessment that is closely in line with the kind of learning experiences in which the students actually engage.

Developing a community-based curriculum

The process of developing a CBE curriculum is labour-intensive and requires the involvement of all stakeholders (academic institution, community and healthcare delivery system) as early as possible. The WHO (1987) recommended that rather than introducing CBE throughout the school at all four levels of the programme, it is better to begin from first year, moving on to second year, while phasing out the old programme. Figure 11.1 outlines the process of planning and implementing a CBE curriculum.

The situational analysis

The situational analysis for a CBE curriculum is directed strongly at the communities targeted as sites, and the health services in such communities. The situational analysis in a community-based curriculum would include:

- information about the gross national product, health expenditure per capita in the area and health indices of mortality and morbidity
- a community profile entailing major demographic characteristics, socio-economic background of the community, norms, culture, habits, traditional health beliefs and practices of the surrounding community, as well as the health status profile of the community
- the type or structure of the healthcare system, its components and proportional distribution of levels of health care
- what are considered as the deficits in graduates' knowledge and skills in meeting their roles in a PHC-oriented healthcare system
- the structure, process, and other factors perceived to be significant for the acquisition of new knowledge required in the transforming healthcare system and nature of nurses required to serve in this type of a healthcare system
- national human resources projections for the present and the future
- education and training capacity of surrounding nursing education institutions and the quality of their education in relation to the needs of the community
- other environmental characteristics and factors that might affect the health of individuals, families and the community (Ezzat, 1995; Nooman, 1989; Refaat et al, 1989).

Identifying, engaging and developing stakeholders

Setting the stage for the innovation and preparing stakeholders for the change is crucial in CBE, because the successful implementation of a CBE curriculum depends on the early involvement of stakeholders (Hamad, 1999). Political commitment of decision-makers is essential when developing a CBE curriculum, as

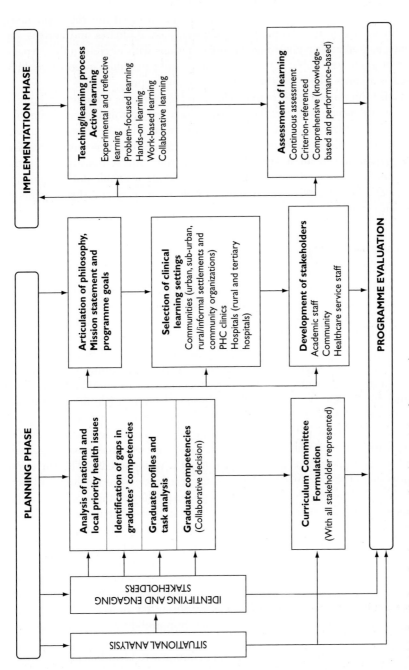

Figure 11.1 Curriculum development and implementation framework

PLANNING PHASE

IMPLEMENTATION PHASE

PROGRAMME EVALUATION

SITUATIONAL ANALYSIS

IDENTIFYING AND ENGAGING STAKEHOLDERS

Analysis of national and local priority health issues

Identification of gaps in graduates' competencies

Graduate profiles and task analysis

Graduate competencies
(Collaborative decision)

Curriculum Committee Formulation
(With all stakeholder represented)

Articulation of philosophy, Mission statement and programme goals

Selection of clinical learning settings
Communities (urban, sub-urban, rural/informal settlements and community organizations)
PHC clinics
Hospitals (rural and tertiary hospitals)

Development of stakeholders
Academic staff
Community
Healthcare service staff

Teaching/learning process
Active learning
Experimental and reflective learning
Problem-focused learning
Hands-on learning
Work-based learning
Collaborative learning

Assessment of learning
Continuous assessment
Criterion-referenced
Comprehensive (knowledge-based and performance-based)

education of this nature demands increased resources, both human and material. Other important stakeholders to be involved are the community, health service sector (hospitals and clinics), past graduates and current students, as well as non-governmental organizations with interest in the preparation of graduates. Public forums, workshops and curriculum meetings could be used as avenues where stakeholders can give their input.

CBE brings a new culture to teaching and learning, as it requires forging of new relationships with healthcare institutions and surrounding communities. Teaching and learning take place in an unfamiliar and unpredictable learning environment (the community), therefore, changing to a new culture requires the preparation of all stakeholders for their roles and responsibilities in this new and unfamiliar education. Stakeholders include academic staff, community members, health service sector staff, as well as students and their parents or significant others.

Teaching staff

CBE depends on the proper preparation of teaching staff as they are regarded as the driving force behind CBE implementation. An effort should be made to ensure a sense of ownership of the proposed change, to secure a spirit of participation and cooperation from the staff. The preparation of the academic staff is, however, a complex task as the new curriculum requires a change in their teaching style, which is like challenging their long cherished beliefs (Irby cited in Hitchcock and Mylona, 2000). The CBE curriculum requires redefinition of relationship with students and other teachers as CBE promotes adult learning principles, student-centred, self-directed and collaborative learning. The change requires teachers to develop an array of skills required in student-centred education, where teachers would be expected to respond to the learners' needs. The preparation of staff should also provide them with essential knowledge, skills and attitudes directly related to the nature of teaching in CBE. The nurse educators should be introduced to the key concepts of the new curriculum (CBE) and be given an opportunity to discuss their understanding of these concepts in the context of the new curriculum. The academic staff should have input in the setting of short- and long-term goals for the innovation being introduced to get their commitment and develop in them ownership of this innovation.

A variety of strategies are recommended in the preparation of academic staff. The staff may be prepared through structured workshops, attending conferences, going for site visits to observe the facilitation of learning in a CBE programme, and inviting experts to assist during the process of change. The academic staff should be prepared for their responsibilities which include:

- leading curriculum transformation in response to identified priority health needs and national policies
- providing expertise regarding community-based educational experiences

- facilitating the learning of students, both in the classroom and community settings
- providing and maintaining appropriate learning resources, and
- ensuring smooth running of the programme.

Health services

The curriculum working committee must approach the healthcare institutions and communities that can provide appropriate learning experiences. Communities and healthcare service staff could also be prepared through meetings and workshops. The healthcare service personnel as well as the community have to be prepared for this new adventure in order to realize their educational potential fully. The healthcare system is developed for the following responsibilities:

- providing a clinical learning environment that is PHC-oriented
- providing personnel to assist in the facilitation of learning in the clinical learning environment
- facilitating learning in the clinical learning environment, and
- sharing of knowledge and expertise on the delivery of comprehensive PHC.

Communities

When developing contact with communities, ideally it is advisable to use academic staff who are familiar with the culture of the community and, if possible, who are known by that community. Once a decision is made about communities to be used, the process of negotiating community entry begins. This is not an easy exercise because of the hierarchy to be observed and respected in the community, as well as the period spent trying to win the trust of some community leaders. Negotiating community entry begins by identifying community leaders. These leaders include people in both formal and informal leadership roles in the community, representing diverse interest groups in the community. These people are usually well informed about everyday events in the community and they keep track of what is happening in the community. The key leaders serve as a very good point of entry to the community as they are very influential in the community. The community needs to be informed about their responsibilities regarding community-based learning experiences. The community is prepared for the following responsibilities:

- providing an environment/context for learning
- facilitating community entry
- ensuring the safety of the students in the community
- providing information that forms part of the curriculum content
- sharing knowledge and skills on handling realities in the community, and

- facilitating some of the learning experiences in the community, which are within their level of expertise (for example, community health workers facilitating home visits).

Students and parents

The preparation of students and parents does not take place during the curriculum planning phase but provision is made at this stage on how they will be prepared for the new programme. Ideally the students' and parents' orientation should take place before the placement of the students in the community settings. This would ensure adequate time to deal with both learners' and parents' concerns. The nursing education institutions might schedule their orientation periods 3–5 weeks before the scheduled university opening time, to avoid clashes with the university's timetable. Workshops or an orientation block could be held with the focus on what CBE is all about, learning in the community, working with people from different groups and cultures in the community, self-directed learning and problem-based learning, learning how to learn, facilitators' and students' roles in CBE, the introduction of basic concepts such as community, community entry, community needs assessment/community survey, health determinants, PHC, epidemiology, community partnerships, group dynamics, transcultural nursing, and many other important issues. Meetings could be held with parents to allay their anxieties regarding the paradigm shift in teaching, the nature of the programme and the nature of the clinical learning environment (community) used.

The academic institution, the community and the healthcare system (three partners) need one another and the expertise of one another to achieve the primary purpose of producing graduates who are competent to serve at all levels of health care. Partnership should be emphasized during the process of preparing these three partners. In such partnership it is believed that there should be mutual respect, joint decision-making and equal power-sharing, with all voices heard equally. In the context of CBE, time and effort spent in the preparation of all stakeholders should be considered as time well invested, because of the need to ensure that all stakeholders participate in and contribute positively to the teaching/learning process.

Defining programme outcomes

The purpose of CBE, which is to achieve educational relevance to the needs of the community, to produce graduates who are responsive to the needs of the population served and contribute in improving the healthcare system, should be expressed in the philosophy, mission statement, goals and programme outcomes.

Defining graduates' competencies should cover a wide range, including primary healthcare competencies, secondary healthcare as well as tertiary healthcare competencies. Programme outcomes of CBE programmes are slightly different from those of traditional hospital programmes. The programme outcomes in a CBE curriculum might be to produce nurses who are able to:

- respond to the health needs and expressed demands of the client by working with the client, in order to stimulate self-determination, self-reliance and healthy living
- address or stimulate action for the solutions of both individual and community health problems
- function independently and collaboratively as members of health teams with a mutual purpose of addressing the client's needs
- take a leadership role completely within a team, in issues requiring nursing expertise
- educate both the community and their co-workers
- continue to learn throughout their work experience, in order to maintain and improve personal competence
- be equipped with the necessary knowledge, skills and attitude to deal with the healthcare problems of urban, suburban, rural and other communities, and adapt that knowledge and skills to other complex situations
- be culturally competent in addressing the health needs of diverse cultural groups in diverse work settings
- be motivated to work in healthcare settings found in under-served or under-developed communities
- be able to function in various teams for the benefit of the client
- be able to contribute towards improving access to quality preventive and promotive health, and quality nursing service to clients of all age groups, and families, at all levels of health care (primary, secondary and tertiary)
- be able to exhibit high levels of professional, ethical and administrative insight, skills and integrity (WHO, 1987).

Collaborative decision making at this stage ensures that the curriculum is acceptable to all stakeholders, is likely to produce competent graduates in terms of stakeholders' needs, and is implementable in the locality where it is supposed to be put into action. Measuring the acceptability and feasibility of a CBE programme is important. According to Jolly and Rees (1998) it is not possible to have a perfect or ideal curriculum, but at least it should meet some general specifications which in their view include: (a) plausibility, (b) fitness for purpose and (c) implementability. Once the basis of the curriculum has been established with the input from all stakeholders, a small working committee (core curriculum committee) is selected. All stakeholders should be represented in this working group to promote ownership of the new curriculum.

Selection of clinical learning settings

The clinical settings selected should be congruent with the wide variety of competencies expected from graduates. In these settings the learners should engage in real-life learning experiences which truly reflect what will be expected from them after graduation. It is crucial to involve the community members as well as representatives from the healthcare system because both these groups know their setting well. More importantly, CBE should take place in a balanced variety of educational settings (primary, secondary and tertiary settings). The primary settings include families, communities, primary healthcare clinics, industries, schools, community-based organizations such as crèches, old age homes, homes for mentally handicapped children, and many more. The secondary healthcare settings include rural and general hospitals, and tertiary institutions include referral healthcare settings, which are more specialized, and use sophisticated technology.

The process of selecting communities as learning sites should begin by defining what is regarded as a community in the context of a particular curriculum or school, as there are multiple interpretations of this term. The WHO (1987) recommends the 'community' be defined geographically in the context of CBE, by using geographic boundaries so that the whole community, across all age groups, benefits from community-based learning experiences, not just a particular group within a community. Special criteria are considered when selecting community learning sites and they include the following:

- ability to provide relevant learning experiences which are in line with the educational outcomes at a particular level
- the presence of community-based organizations, including PHC clinics, that can serve as bases while students are placed in the community. These organizations should believe in PHC, which should be the philosophy underlying their activities
- stability and safety
- need of service (in under-served communities) that will be provided by the students during their community-based learning experiences
- the feasibility of organizing community-based education activities depends on the possibility of collaborating with the local healthcare human resources, accessibility, and affordability of transport to be used by the students, accommodation where necessary and many other factors. Feasibility is the key aspect when selecting community learning sites
- diversity of population, to expose students to diverse cultures and rich experiences associated with different cultures
- range from rural, suburban to urban communities, including informal settlements, to expose students to a variety of rich learning experiences
- other disciplines using that community to expose students to multidisciplinary learning

- ability to provide a number of community services, including schools, police stations, day care centres, food establishments/shops, businesses, churches or place of worship, social services, health services, etc.

The nature of community-based learning experiences

Community-based learning experiences in CBE have a strong primary health-care focus with the purpose of socializing students to PHC. Therefore the selected community learning sites should allow for the following learning experiences:

- conducting a home visit and a family study
- conducting a community survey and playing an active role in planning, implementing and evaluating an action plan which is aimed at addressing one, or some, of the identified community health problems
- participating in health promotion and illness prevention learning activities
- working in a variety of community settings with the intention of providing service and at the same time conceptualizing how psychosocial, economic, cultural and political factors affect the health of individuals, families and communities (Hamad, 2000)
- conducting an epidemiological study.

The curriculum committee has to revisit the competencies required from the programme and plans how these competencies can be developed. Table 11.1 outlines the competencies required that might be expected from graduates and the tasks that will facilitate the development of that expected competence.

Implementing a community-based curriculum

The teaching/learning process

Experiential learning theory is regarded as the main theory underpinning the learning process in CBE. The learning process follows Kolb's four-staged cycle: concrete experience, reflective observation, abstract conceptualization and active experimentation as shown in Figure 11.2. The teaching/learning process begins by exposing students to concrete experiences, where students immerse themselves fully and openly in new experiences in the clinical learning settings (for example, conducting a community survey).

The most commonly used CBE teaching/learning approaches, both in the classroom and in clinical learning settings, facilitate active learning, learning through experience and reflection, self-directed learning and collaborative learning. Active learning as stated in Della-Dora and Wells (2001) refers to learning where students move away from being passive recipients of knowledge, to being active participants doing most of the work, learning through experience,

Table 11.1 Community-based tasks linked to competencies to be achieved

Competence	Task
Develop a community profile	• Do area mapping • Conduct a windshield survey to assess the available resources, infrastructure in the community, to establish history of the community and observe different socio-cultural and religious patterns and practices in the community, as well as to identify social problems and health needs of the community • Formulate a community diagnosis • Compile a report of the findings
Formulate, a plan for a community intervention programme, implement and evaluate it in partnership with the community, members of the multidisciplinary team and other sectors in the community	• Review a community profile with the focus on social problems and data on health and disease patterns in that community • Validate the identified needs and problems within the community project • Solicit the involvement of other sectors and community members in the development of an integrated plan for the community • Research possible intervention strategies • Select one intervention which is more appropriate and which is implementable (taking into consideration the cost implications, time, and other required resources) • Develop a proposal for the intervention programme, including the budget • Raise funds for the intervention programme • Implementing a community intervention • Research appropriate programme evaluation strategies and select one strategy • Evaluate an intervention programme including community partnership or community involvement • Report on the whole process, starting from the planning phase to the evaluation phase (orally or in writing).

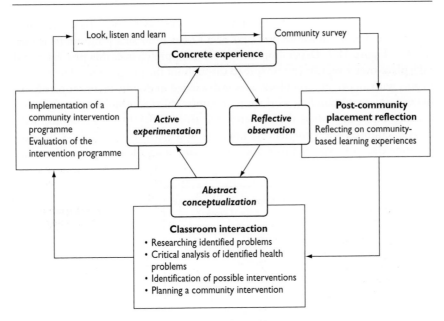

Figure 11.2 Experiential learning cycle in community-based learning

engaging in problem-solving activities and knowledge-construction exercises, as well as in the application of what has been learned, with teachers facilitating and directing the process of learning.

Learning through reflection is also encouraged, as experiential learning and problem-focused approaches are the main approaches used. The reflection process provides students with an opportunity to think about and interpret their experiences in the clinical learning settings. They have an opportunity to share their knowledge and understanding of their experiences with one another, noting ways in which their learning experiences were meaningful to them (Lankard, 1998). They also do self-assessment, identifying gaps in their knowledge and acting on those gaps as self-directed learners. Promotion of reflective learning is one way of trying to develop reflective practitioners. Collaborative learning is also promoted in CBE, where students learn in groups. Learning in groups prepares them for their professional roles where they will be working in teams. They have an opportunity to develop skills required when working in teams and facilitate the understanding of different personalities encountered in real-life settings.

An example

The following section presents an example of a pathway followed in one nursing education institution (University of KwaZulu-Natal, South Africa) which is based on Kolb's experiential learning cycle. The community-based learning experience (CBLE) in the second year of a 4-year B-nursing programme is outlined in Figure 11.3. Depending on the school's preference, this process could take place over 1 year or can be spread throughout the programme. The process begins with an orientation block as was discussed under the preparation of students and a team-building workshop or camp. This team-building workshop is crucial, especially when the students are from different backgrounds, with diverse cultures, life experiences, interests and personalities. In a CBE programme they are expected to work very closely in small teams. The diversities

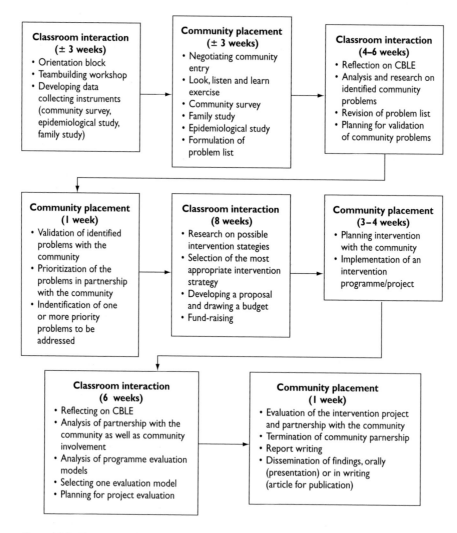

Figure 11.3 Community-based learning process

within a group, if not positively utilized, impact on the students' effectiveness in the community. The team-building exercise should aim at preparing students for the immediate application of skills learned and the future application of those skills when functioning in multidisciplinary and intersectoral teams. The orientation block also entails preparing students for the assessment phase of the community-based learning experiences. This includes developing data-collecting instruments for conducting community surveys, home visits, family studies, nutritional assessments and epidemiological studies. The students prepare these instruments under the guidance of the facilitator. The ability to develop instruments for data collection is one competence required from a CBE graduate, where research is emphasized. The orientation block might take about 3 weeks or more depending on the time available.

Once the tools have been developed and approved by the facilitators, the students are placed in groups in a variety of under-served community settings, some in an urban community, some in a suburban community and others in a rural community or an informal settlement. Placing students in different settings helps them understand the diversity of problems in communities. Learning experiences during the first community placement include a look, listen and learn exercise, walking or driving around the community, doing observations, listening to conversations, noise from the environment and learning whatever is there to learn.

This exercise takes place on the first day in the community and is rounded off by a session where students reflect on what they have observed, heard and learned from the community. After walking around the community, a decision is made about the boundaries demarcating the area which will be used for learning experiences in that particular year, especially if the community is too big to be managed by a small group of students. The students can use the first day or the second day for identifying key figures and making appointments to meet them or they can do that on the second day in the community. The purpose of identifying and meeting the key figures is to develop in the students the ability to negotiate community entry. The students might interview key figures or conduct community meetings to learn more about the community values, beliefs, health and cultural practices as well as health needs. The formulation of a community needs or problems list is crucial because what appears on that list forms part of the curriculum content in that particular year.

In CBE, learning in the classrooms is highly influenced by what is happening in the community settings. In the classroom there is translation of community-based learning experiences and meaning is made out of those experiences. The process begins by reflecting on community-based learning experiences to establish what was learned, to identify gaps in students' knowledge and to plan on how the identified gaps will be addressed. The identified community needs and problems are tabled in class and a plan is made about how they will be dealt with in class. The students conduct a thorough literature review of these problems to give classroom discussion a scientific or theoretical basis. The process of analysing community problems might take a long time, 4–6 weeks with students meeting twice a week for about two lecture-periods a day. Once all problems have been analysed a new list is formulated with the priority problems, according to the students' view, listed as first on the list. This list of community problems/needs compiled by the students is subjected to the scrutiny of the community during the second community placement of students. The community validates if the list has prevalent problems in that particular community and then prioritizes these problems according to how they view them in the community. Community meetings, interviews or structured questionnaires could be used to obtain data from the community. Once validation and prioritization is done, a decision by the community in partnership with the students is made about priority problem(s) to be addressed, taking feasibility into consideration.

Preparations for addressing the identified problem(s) take place during the following classroom sessions. This course is focused on health promotion and therefore students are required to identify a health promotion project, and not a treatment of care project. The students study the relevant health promotion strategies and invite experts from other disciplines or sectors if there is a need, to share their expertise with them. For example, if the students plan to start a vegetable garden as an income generating project, they can invite an expert from the agriculture department to do the soil analysis, advise the students about soil preparation before planting, the types of vegetables that will grow well in that particular soil, how to grow and care for those vegetables. The students can also invite an expert from the economics department at the university to teach them about handling of finances in an income-generating project. Community interventions may range from the clean-up campaigns, health awareness campaigns (HIV/AIDS awareness, teenage pregnancy, child abuse, drug and alcohol abuse), skills development and income generating projects such as sewing, chicken farming, bricklaying, gardening, baking and selling and many more.

One health promotion strategy out of the many identified is selected, and a proposal as well as the budget for the community intervention is developed. The students start raising funds by seeking sponsorships for the project. These preparations might take up to 6 weeks or more. Thereafter the intervention programme is implemented with the community playing an active role and students facilitating the process. Classroom interactions following the implementation of a community programme entail planning for the evaluation of a project, researching various programme evaluation strategies and selecting the most appropriate one. Plans for data collection are made during class time, developing data collecting instruments (questionnaires and interview guides) and/or planning community meetings where necessary. The last community placement is used to evaluate the community-based learning experiences and the impact in that particular community. That opportunity is also used to terminate the partnership with the community or to hand them over to a community organization that will continue working with the community on the initiated project. The partnership-terminating phase is the challenging phase because the two partners (community and students) will have developed some special bonds during their working relationships and severing these ties is emotional and challenging to the community and the students. The students are advised to start preparing the community partners for termination from the beginning of their community placement and throughout the year.

Once the data have been collected for evaluation they are analysed and findings are communicated through the evaluation report. The students may write an article for publication to share their learning experiences with the larger public. A special day may also be organized by the school in which the students can publicly share their community learning experiences with the other members of the school, the invited community members from the different clinical learning sites, parents, new recruits to the school and the university community at large.

During the course of CBE, a problem-solving process is followed with hands-on learning through experience. The students learn to identify and work towards solving the identified problems in partnership with clients. They learn research skills including developing instruments for data analysis, collecting data, analyse data statistically and qualitatively and disseminate their findings either verbally or in writing.

Assessment of learning in community-based education

Assessment in a community-based curriculum poses a challenge, because traditional methods of assessment are usually not relevant to assessing learning that is community-based. Therefore plans for evaluation should be made during the planning phase, including developing instruments for assessing learning. Continuous assessment and criterion-referenced assessment are favoured in CBE.

Magzoub et al. (1998) recommended a comprehensive approach to student assessment because the assessment of this nature gives a holistic picture of learning that has taken place with three domains (cognitive, affective and psychomotor) taken into consideration. This comprehensive approach incorporates three main approaches to assessment:

- performance-based
- knowledge measurement approach, and
- the comprehensive approach, which brings together the other approaches.

Knowledge measurement uses pen and paper methods which assess factual recall and in some cases knowledge application. Knowledge measurement is characteristically conducted at the end of a community-based activity. Tools applied in measuring knowledge are essays, reports, tests and examinations. Performance-based approaches mainly assess the performance of students during their field activities, through observational methods. The performance-based approach assesses all domains required in a competence being assessed. A wide range of tools are used in performance assessment including logbooks, learning contracts, reflective learning diaries, supervisory visits, peer assessment, community leaders' feedback, mentoring and monitoring of attendance. Each assessment method focuses on specific aspects of the community-based programme. Magzoub et al. (1998) appraising a comprehensive approach to assessment, asserted that it is sensitive to the objectives of CBE and enhances the production of health professionals who are more likely to be responsive to the health needs of the community. It is appropriate because it measures the various competencies needed in the context of CBE; it takes into consideration not only the impact of community-based learning on the students but also on the community. The community also participates in the assessment of the students. They have an input regarding community participation or involvement, impact of the service provided by the students and the observation of nursing values while working in and with the community. Although comprehensive assessment is recommended in CBE, it is very time-consuming and requires assessors who are familiar with innovative teaching strategies.

Conclusion

Developing and implementing a community-based curriculum is a labour-intensive exercise and requires adhering to the CBE principles. CBE programmes might vary from institution to institution because of the influence of the surrounding community and the needs of the local healthcare services. CBE promotes the personal, social, psychological and intellectual development of the student. It heightens the sense of personal and social responsibility, develops a positive attitude towards serving in under-resourced rural community settings which have been in the past severely affected by poor staff retention. Personally the students develop a number of life skills which are transferable, such as complex patterns of thinking, problem-solving abilities, communication skills, and their mastery of skills and content is directly related to practice.

Points for discussion

1. How can one deal with the issue of the safety of students when they go into under-served communities?
2. Is this curriculum approach more relevant in developing countries than in developed countries? Why do you think so?

References

Al-Refai, A. M. (1995) Exploring models of cooperation. *Medical Education*, **29**(1): 53–55.

Della-Dora, D. and Wells, J. D. (2001) Teaching for self-directed learning. **XIX**(2): 134–140.

Ezzat, E. (1995) Role of the community in contemporary health professions education. *Medical Education*, **29**(1): 44–52.

Hamad, B. (1999) Establishing community-oriented medical schools: Key issues and steps in early planning. *Medical Education*, **33**: 382–389.

Hamad, B. (2000) What is community-based education? Evolution, definition and rationale. In: H. G. Schmidt, M. Magzoub, G. Felletti, Z. H. Nooman and S. Vluggen. *Handbook on Community-based Education*, pp. 11–26. Maastrich: Network Publications.

Hitchcock, M. A and Mylona, Z. A. (2000) 'Special article' – Teaching faculty to conduct PBL. *Teaching and Learning in Medicine*, **12**(1): 52–57.

Jolly, B. and Rees, L. (1998). *Medical Education in the Millennium*. New York: Oxford University Press.

Lankard, B. (1998) New learning for generation X. ERIC Digest No. 184. http://www.ericdigest.org/1998-1/x.htm (accessed 26 January 2005).

Magzoub, M. A., Schmidt, H. G., Abdel-Hameed, A. A., Dolmans, D. and Mustafa, S. E. (1998) Student assessment in community-settings: a comprehensive approach. *Medical Education*, **32**: 50–59.

McWhinney, I. R. (1980) The reform in medical education: a Canadian model. *Medical Education*, **14**: 189–195.

Nooman, Z. M. (1989) Implementation of community-oriented curriculum: The tasks and the problems. In H. G. Schmidt, M. Lipkin, M. de Vries and J. M. Greep (eds) *New Directions for Medical Education: Problem-based Learning and Community-oriented Medical Education*, pp. 66–77. London: Springer-Verlag.

Quinn, S. C., Gamble, D. and Denham, A. (2000) Ethics and community-based education: Balancing respect for the community with professional preparation. *Family Community Health*, **23**(4): 9–23

Refaat, A. H., Nooman, Z. M. and Richards, R. W. (1989) A model for planning a community-based medical school curriculum. *Annals of Community-Oriented Education*, **2**: 7–18.

World Health Organization (1985) *Health Manpower Requirements for the Achievement of Health for All by the Year 2000 through Primary Health Care*. WHO Technical Report Series 717. Geneva: WHO.

World Health Organization (1987) *Community-based Education of Health Personnel*. Report of the WHO Study Group. Technical Report Series No. 746. Geneva: WHO.

World Health Organization (1993) *Increasing the Relevance of Education for Health Professionals*. Report of WHO study group on problem solving education for health professionals. WHO Technical Report Series 838. Geneva: WHO.

Recommended reading

Examples of schools running community-based education programmes

University of Central Florida

Source: Mattesson, P. S. (2000) *Community-based Nursing Education: The Experience of Eight Schools*. New York: Springer Publishing Company.

The School of Nursing at the University of KwaZulu-Natal, in Durban, the World Health Organization's (WHO's) Collaborating Centre for Nursing and Midwifery Development in Africa. Website: http://www.ukzn.ac.za.

Chapter 12

Developing an outcomes-based curriculum

Ntombifikile G Mtshali

Introduction

Outcomes-based education (OBE) is a competency-oriented, performance-based approach to education which is aimed at aligning education with the demands of the workplace, and at the same time develops transferable life skills, such as problem-solving and critical-thinking skills. A paradigm shift to OBE came about as a result of its potential to address the concerns about graduates from conventional nursing programmes. Some of these concerns include that newly employed graduates come to clinical settings academically equipped, yet with limited ability to apply their knowledge. Their mastery of life skills (such as, problem solving skills, leadership skills, communication skills, critical-thinking skills) required in contemporary clinical environments, is limited. They struggle to cope with the dynamics in clinical settings. Professionals in healthcare settings find themselves helping these graduates make the transition from being students to being professional practitioners. Employing such graduates has many legal and financial implications in the workplace or healthcare system with the institutions having to spend time and money during the first years of practice of such practitioners to get them up to speed.

Another motivation for the move to OBE is that this approach allows for the recognition of prior learning, and transfer of credits, thus avoiding unnecessary duplication of learning. This chapter is divided into two sections, the understanding of outcomes-based education and the process of developing an outcomes-based curriculum.

Understanding the concept of outcomes-based education

An analysis of the concept of OBE reveals a wide range in the understanding of this term. OBE is sometimes used interchangeably with the terms competency-based education and performance-based education. In the context of this chapter, OBE will be defined as an approach to education in which decisions about the curriculum are driven by the outcomes the learners should demonstrate on completion of the programme, with the product defining the process. The educational outcomes are clearly specified from the beginning of the programme and decisions about content and how it is organized, educational strategies, teaching methods, assessment procedures and the educational environment are made in the context of the stated learning outcomes (Harden et al., 1999). OBE organizes the whole educational system around what is essential for the students to be able to do successfully at the end of the learning experiences (Spady, 1994).

The term outcome

In OBE, the term 'outcome' is regarded as the core concept. This term is sometimes used interchangeably with the terms 'competency', 'standards', 'benchmarks' and 'attainment targets'. An outcome is a statement of what a learner is expected to be able to do (demonstrate) as a result of the learning process. In the words of Spady:

> Outcomes are clear, observable demonstrations of student learning that occur at or after the end of a significant set of learning experiences. . . . . Typically, these demonstrations, or performances reflect three key things: (1) what the student knows, (2) what the student can actually DO with what he or she knows, and (3) the student's confidence and motivation in carrying out the demonstration. A well defined outcome will have clearly defined content or concepts and a well defined demonstration process – like "explain", "organize", "produce" (1994: 20, 21).

According to Spady, 'demonstration' is the key word in the term 'outcome', with learners demonstrating in terms of knowledge, skills and values or attitudes what they are able to do, on completion of a clearly defined learning process. A variety of outcomes are reported in OBE and these include critical outcomes, programme outcomes, exit level outcomes, specific area outcomes, unit outcomes and lesson/lecture outcomes.

Outcomes-based education approaches

Spady (1994a) analysed a number of OBE programmes and suggested three approaches to OBE: traditional, transitional and transformational. Authors such as Bonville (1996) view these three approaches as different stages the schools might undergo in the process of implementing an outcomes-based programme. As schools get familiar with OBE, they gradually move to a transformational approach. The understanding of these types of OBE could be helpful in evaluating the existing OBE programmes in different schools.

Traditional OBE shares some characteristics with objectives- or content-based education. It retains the focus on traditional subject area knowledge, with the purpose of producing academically competent graduates. Outcomes are used to focus and align the existing subjects. The curriculum content is discipline-specific, with no integration of subjects. The outcomes are drawn directly from the content of an existing syllabus, which is used to direct instruction. The focus in this type of OBE is on mastery of small sections of the content or discrete skills in little steps, with no clear picture of long-term outcomes of learning or of how different objectives relate to each other or society. The teacher, however, takes the role of a facilitator, facilitating the learning process. A criterion-referenced approach rather than a normative approach is used in the assessment of learning.

Although traditional OBE may improve the learners' learning, traditional OBE has a number of limitations, including:

- It does not give learners or educators an understanding of why this learning is important.
- It focuses strongly on either doing or recalling content: it does not focus on linking or integrating skills, knowledge and values. This integration is essential to operate competently in an ever-changing society.
- Because of this education, educators do not change the learning environment much – things carry on just as they did before the outcomes were defined. So, while teaching and learning may be more clearly focused, traditional OBE is unlikely to transform the school completely (Department of Education, 1997a).

Transitional OBE is also centred around academic subject areas, but is more focused on the development of cross-disciplinary skills and qualities that the learners need to function competently in the society. The main question asked in transitional OBE is 'Why do learners need to know this?' This question serves to establish the relevance of what is being learned to the needs of the learner or society. Critical outcomes serve as the point of departure when developing a transitional OBE curriculum. Transitional OBE incorporates the characteristics of traditional OBE and those of transformational OBE. Traditional OBE is more visible during the curriculum development process and transformational OBE is more marked during the teaching/learning process with the intention of orientating the learners to their future role (Spady and Marshall, 1991). Transitional OBE uses alternative methods of assessment and the grading system, for instance portfolios, instead of relying on traditional examinations.

The following differences exist between transitional and traditional OBE. In transitional OBE:

- Planning begins with critical outcomes and the content is simply used to achieve these outcomes and not the other way round.
- Educators always ask whether the outcomes have any value to society as opposed to simply being useful within teaching and learning or simply being chosen by educators on the basis of their perceived intrinsic value.

- There is a distinct focus on integrating knowing, doing and feeling, as opposed to focusing on each domain separately.

The limitations of transitional OBE include that irrelevant content remains in the curriculum, just as in a traditional approach, and that although creative ways of teaching are used, some of the old practices such as the use of the lecture method may still dominate (Department of Education, 1997a).

Transformational OBE arises from the conviction that the existing education system and syllabus impede the development of a new society and do not help learners to develop the attitude, knowledge and skills that will enable them to participate competently in the competitive global community. The premise of this type of OBE is that the education system should be transformed in order to produce competent future citizens who can contribute to the realization of a transformed society. Transformational OBE places emphasis on the demonstration of complex applications of many kinds of competencies (knowledge, skills and attitudes) as people confront the challenges surrounding them in their social systems (Spady, 1994). Transformational OBE focuses on the competence of learners to perform the roles demanded by their future 'high tech' and competitive professional lives.

The sole determinants of the curriculum in transformational OBE are critical outcomes. The curriculum planning process, including the input as well as the process, is directed by the critical outcomes, thus facilitating a design-down process of curriculum development. This approach requires that teaching directly relate to the local context and that the curriculum changes rapidly when changes in society and in the workplace demands it. More importantly, success at school (or any other learning) is considered to be of limited benefit unless learners are equipped to transfer that success to life beyond the school. The student should also see learning as a lifelong process, which is essential to keep pace with rapidly changing conditions in the world of work and in society. Transformational OBE is the type of OBE implemented in a number of countries such as New Zealand, Australia, South Africa, and the UK because of its reform oriented focus.

Characteristics of transformational OBE

OBE, just like all approaches to education, has core characteristics which include the following:

- The OBE curriculum is informed by the professional or workplace expectations (specific knowledge, skills and attitudes needed for entry level into the world of work); the general knowledge, skills and attitudes (transferable core skills such as problem solving, collecting, analysing and organizing information) needed for entry level to the world of work; and current and future trends in the workplace (e.g. dynamics in the workplace and society).

- What the learner needs to learn is clearly and unambiguously stated from the beginning of the programme and is followed throughout the learning process.
- The learner is facilitated towards the achievement of the outcomes (by the teacher, who acts as a facilitator rather than a mere presenter or conveyor of knowledge), with the learner being an active and interested participant in the learning process.
- The learner's progress is based on his or her demonstrated achievement. The focus is on being able to use and apply learned knowledge, skills and attitude, rather than on merely absorbing specific and prescribed bodies of content.
- Continuous assessment functions as a tool to help learners learn through experience using authentic learning experiences, with the facilitator facilitating their learning.
- Each learner's needs are catered for by means of a variety of instructional strategies and assessment tools.
- Applied competence is emphasized in OBE with the learners demonstrating their ability to perform tasks with understanding and to adapt learnt behaviour to new situations. Applied competence is further broken down to practical competence (demonstration or ability to do something), foundational competence (understanding or demonstrating ability to describe what one is doing theoretically and why one is doing that in a particular way) and 'reflexive competence' (the ability to pass judgement on a course of action and give reasoned argument on how it could be done differently or better where appropriate).

Developing an outcomes-based curriculum

Outcomes-based education uses a design-down approach in developing a curriculum. The process of developing a curriculum begins with a clear specification of what the students should know, be able to do and the attitudes desirable on completion of the programme. The curriculum process in OBE entails the following steps:

1. developing a graduate role statement (see Chapter 4)
2. determining graduate competencies in the form of programme outcomes
3. deciding on the programme structure, ensuring that all outcomes are catered for in the programme
4. identification and designing of modules/course outlines
5. planning the assessment and evaluation of learning.

Determining graduate competencies

Determining graduate competencies requires identification of graduates' tasks and expected competencies in performing particular tasks and determining elements of each competency. The term competence in OBE is not limited to skills only, but incorporates knowledge, skills and values to be demonstrated by graduates when performing a task. Research is conducted on tasks performed by the graduates in clinical settings and these tasks are explicitly defined so that one is able to analyse them to show the knowledge, skills, attitudes and values expected in each task. The information about the tasks performed by the graduates can be obtained from the graduates, employers of the graduates, experienced practitioners, surrounding community members and students. The graduates might be asked to indicate their core problem areas in practice, as well as key competencies required in practice. The curriculum planners should start by defining exactly what the job of the graduate entails and what the graduates are expected to do (tasks) in that particular job. Prozesky (2003) suggested that one could (a) observe health professionals at work and write down what they did every day, (b) conduct interviews with health professionals themselves regarding the tasks they perform every day, (c) consult official documents, such as job descriptions for that category of health professionals, and (d) look at the available health statistics and work out what the health professional should be able to do.

Over and above the analysis of tasks, discussions should be held with the management or authorities of the institutions regarding their future plans, so that it can be established what type of graduate might contribute to the success of the institution. For example, the healthcare institutions are gradually moving towards the use of computers or information technology for data management. This could be one area to be addressed in a new competency-oriented curriculum.

It is important to note that some of the tasks may share some common elements. This should be taken into consideration when planning the modules and learning experiences to avoid unnecessary duplication in teaching and learning. Once the exercise of analysing tasks is completed, a competency profile for the graduates should be constructed and sent back to the experts in the clinical field and to those involved in teaching, for validation purposes. Competencies in a competency profile may be categorized according to the different roles of the graduate, the clinical, professional, management, leadership and research roles, as indicated below.

In countries with comprehensive pre-registration nursing programmes, the clinical role can be further divided according to special areas, such as general nursing, community health nursing, mental health nursing and midwifery. Professionals and discipline experts should be requested to rate competencies according to their importance in the discipline, and how frequently those competencies are required in practice. The rating of competencies assists in making decisions about crucial areas in the preparation of graduates.

Example of graduate roles

A. Clinical role
- Assess comprehensively the health needs of clients using appropriate technology, in order to make relevant and accurate diagnoses.
- Develop a care plan in collaboration with the client, and/or team based on relevant information.

B. Management role
- Manage a healthcare unit effectively by planning, organizing, supervising and evaluating the functioning of the unit.

C. Research role
- Gather and analyse information about practice, management and professional problems.
- Develop a proposal for work-based research, which includes a budget.

D. Clinical teaching role
- Facilitate the learning of students in the clinical areas through coaching, supervision, role modelling and assessment.

Developing programme outcomes

Programme outcomes are those outcomes which should be demonstrated by learners when they have completed a programme. Based on the role statement, programme outcomes or capabilities are identified and defined. When formulating an outcome it should include three elements:

- an observable behaviour which will demonstrate that the student knows specified content and/or can apply/use knowledge
- the conditions under which the student must perform the behaviour and
- the criteria against which the performance will be measured.

Example of an outcome: The students accurately record (behaviour) health practices of adolescent clients giving reasons in terms of beliefs and knowledge (criterion) without using a computer software program (condition).

There is not a set number of programme outcomes. They are likely to vary as determined by the needs of the programme.

Example: A pre-registration nursing programme outcome

On successful completion of this programme, the graduate will be able to:

- Conduct a comprehensive and appropriate assessment of the health status of a client of any age, presenting with any level of health or disease, using appropriate technology, in order to make relevant and accurate diagnoses.
- Develop a plan of action (nursing care plan or treatment plan) in collaboration with the client and/or members of the multidisciplinary team, based on a relevant assessment and accurate diagnosis.
- Implement a health promotion/illness prevention programme in collaboration with a group or community.
- Provide appropriate treatment and care to mentally or physically ill individuals of all ages, in PHC and secondary healthcare settings.

Developing a programme structure for the curriculum

The structure of the programme involves decisions about the fundamental modules, core modules and elective modules required in a particular qualification, as well as the organization of the curriculum according to different levels in a programme. Fundamental modules provide basic contents upon which the rest of the programme builds, for example in a pre-registration nursing programme, social sciences, foundational sciences such as anatomy, physiology and many other modules may be regarded as fundamental modules. Core modules provide compulsory learning required in situations contextually relevant to the particular qualification, for instance, for a nursing programme, nursing courses will be core modules.

Elective modules are those modules which can be selected for additional credits. These modules could be chosen to enrich the programme or to develop learners in specific areas.

In OBE it is emphasized that programmes should not be a dead end. They should make provision for those learners who cannot complete the course of study for some reason, by building in multiple exit points for the learners to earn some recognition in the form of a diploma or certificate, for the work they have done. Flexible exit and entry points contribute to the attractiveness of programmes for prospective learners.

A curriculum should be structured so that different levels in the programme are identified. This structuring of the curriculum allows for the identification level of outcomes and modules to be taken at each level. The organization depends on the duration of the programme. The pre-registration nursing programme may run over 3 or 4 years. Table 12.1 shows how a comprehensive

Table 12.1 Possible levels in a 4-year comprehensive programme

Programme level	Option 1	Option 2
1	Fundamental nursing: Competencies with regard to basic needs Placement: crèche, old age home, hospitals	The nursing process: Competencies of assessment and planning for individuals and groups Placement: PHC services, school, health services
2	General nursing: Competencies with regard to different body systems Placement: Hospitals	Nursing interventions: Competencies with regard to different problems of individuals and groups Placement: Hospitals and other institutions
3	Community health nursing: Competencies with regard to aggregate care Placement: Community health care settings (PHC clinics)	Maternal and child health care (midwifery) Competencies in maternal and child health care (primary health care) Placement: Maternal and child healthcare services
4	Maternal and child health care (midwifery) Competencies in maternal and child health care (midwife) Placement: Maternal and child healthcare services	Mental health nursing (Psychiatry) Competencies in mental health care services. Placement: Mental health care services (in the community, primary and tertiary healthcare settings)

pre-registration nursing programme can be planned over a period of 4 years. This table has two options. The first level in the programme can be organized so that fundamental courses/modules are taken at this level and they are used as a foundation to build on.

When a curriculum is built around outcomes, these outcomes should be formulated in a way that structures the teaching/learning process adequately. This is particularly true about module outcomes, which should be quite specific to direct the choices of learning experiences and assessment methods. To achieve this clarity the outcome statement itself should adhere to specific criteria, but each module outcome may also be augmented with a range of clarifying statements which defines it more specifically. A comprehensive outcome statement is given in Table 12.2 to illustrate the outcome statement and its clarifying statements.

Table 12.2 An example of a module outcome with clarifying statements

Level 1 outcome: *The learner should be able to assess the health, the health behaviour, physical and mental status of individuals of any age.*
Range statement: Psychiatric assessment of a child is not expected from a nurse with preregistration training only.

Specific outcome	*Assessment criteria*
The learners will:	
Assess the health behaviours and underlying knowledge and beliefs of an adult with regard to the client's own basic needs	The assessment data are comprehensive and accurate, they include information related to health practices of the adult and reasons are given in terms of beliefs and knowledge. The assessment is in accordance with verifiable standard texts
Assess the health behaviour and underlying knowledge and beliefs of adults caring for children and the elderly with regard to the basic needs of clients	Health practices of adult carers are accurately recorded and motivation behind the health practices is in terms of beliefs and knowledge found in standard health assessment text
Take a complete history from an adult or a child in terms of physical and mental health of the client	History obtained from a client is accurate and complete, it includes a chief complaint, history of the present illness, past history and family or social history. Obtained history is accurately documented in accordance with institutional guidelines
Perform a physical examination of an adult or a child	A detailed and accurate physical examination is performed within a set time limit and according to the standard protocol used. The results of a completed physical examination of an adult or child are accurately and briefly recorded, taking into consideration principles observed when recording patient data
Conduct a mental status examination of an adult	A detailed and accurate mental status examination of an adult client is performed according to acceptable institutional guidelines and/or standard text. The results of a mental examination of an adult are accurately recorded following the institutional guidelines for recording data

Specific outcomes

These are outcomes at a micro-curriculum or module level, which define context-specific competencies that learners must demonstrate at the end of every module. Every statement of specific outcomes should be derived from and should contribute towards the attainment of exit level outcomes. In writing specific outcomes, it is recommended that one complete the phrase 'learners will . . .' by adding both a verb and a noun, for instance 'Learners will administer medication'.

Range statements

These statements describe the scope, depth and level of complexity and parameter of the achievement. The range statements include critical areas of content, processes and context which the learners should engage with in order to reach the acceptable level of competence but does not restrict learning to specific lists of knowledge items or activities which learners can work through mechanically. It provides direction, allows for multiple learning strategies and flexibility in the choice of specific content and process and for a variety of assessment methods. For instance, a range statement for the administration of medication might include:

- Scope: Orally, parentally, and rectally, but not intravenously.
- Content: Within legal requirements, with the ability to anticipate possible side-effects.

Example of a range statement

This course/module provides the nurse with fundamental knowledge, skills and attitudes required when assessing the health of individuals of any age, enabling him/her to assess comprehensively the client or carers of clients. This module however does not prepare nurses for psychiatric assessment of a child, as this skill is not expected from a nurse in a pre-registration programme.

Assessment criteria

These statements provide evidence that the learner has achieved the specific outcome. To distinguish between the outcome statement and the assessment criteria, it is useful to commence every assessment criterion statement with a noun, describing the product of the action described in the outcome (see examples in Table 12.2). The assessment criteria indicate in broad terms, the observable processes and products of learning which serve as culminating demonstrations of learners' achievement or competence.

It is important to note that assessment criteria are supposed to be broadly stated so that they do not themselves provide sufficient details of exactly what and how much learning marks an acceptable level of the outcome. They provide a framework for assessment, not a detailed description of what exactly is expected to make a decision that the learner is competent.

The process of developing outcomes and the assessment criteria is the same in all stages in the OBE curriculum, starting from the programme outcomes, to level outcomes, module outcomes and unit outcomes.

The specific outcomes in a module can be achieved through a set of units within a module. The process of identifying specific outcomes and their assessment criteria is then followed by the designing of a course or module outline which includes units that will contribute towards achieving the specific outcomes. Figure 12.1 illustrates the process followed when developing a curriculum from the level outcome down to the unit outcomes. The level outcome is achieved through a number of modules which are also made up of a number of units. All these are linked contributing to the level outcomes as well as programme outcomes.

Unlike traditional education, OBE does not follow the content of a textbook or a traditional syllabus. The educators, guided by specific outcomes, have the responsibility to decide what content is important, what the relevant and effective teaching methods are and which forms of assessment are appropriate to guide the learners to meet the set outcomes. The term module is usually used in OBE curricula and refers to a self-contained component, often built around a specific competency or set of competencies which form a coherent whole and which are separately assessed. It is built on the assumption that formal learning

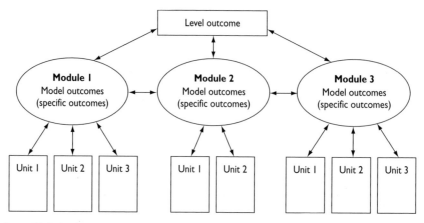

Figure 12.1 An illustration of the relationship between units, modules and level outcomes.

can be broken into self-contained blocks (modules) in which students can learn and then show through assessment that they have attained a competence.

The modules in a programme and units within a module are supposed to be presented in a logical sequence to promote meaningful learning, with the foundational units presented first to lay a foundation for the subsequent units (see Table 12.3 showing the organization of units in a 'nursing assessment course or module'). There are five units making up the module in the example in Table 12.3, each addressing a specific competence or outcome.

The course outline (micro-curriculum) should stipulate the expected learning outcomes for the course or module, the content to be covered in each unit, teaching/learning methods to be used, clinical placement and directives for what the learner should do in that clinical setting (learning experience) as indicated in Table 12.3.

Table 12.3 The outline for a nursing assessment course

Outcomes and content	Teaching/learning methods	Clinical placement and directives
1. Assessment of health behaviour of adult 1.1 Health behaviour 1.2 Interviewing 1.3 Observation 1.4 Basic needs	Lecture on 1.1 and 1.4 Demonstration, reading and discussion on 1.3 Role play of 1.2 Workbook; total procedure	Interviews with hospitalized adults Home visits to families Task: Do assessment
2. Assess caring for vulnerable groups 2.1 Institutionalized people 2.2 Refugees	Readings on 2.1 and 2.2 Workbook	Family visit to refugee family Visits to care facility for elderly Task: Do assessment
3. History taking 3.1 Structure of history interview 3.2 Components of interview 3.3 Parameters of variables 3.4 Dealing with problems in interview	Reading on 3.2, 3.3 and 3.4 Demonstration and role playing 3.1 and 3.4 Video vignettes 3.3	Outpatient department Inpatient units Home visits to clients with chronic conditions Task: Take histories
4. Physical examination 4.1 Using different instruments 4.2 Organization of examination 4.3 Normal vs. abnormal findings 4.4 Adaptations with different age groups 4.5 Psychosocial aspects	Demonstration 4.1 Readings on 4.2, 4.3 and 4.4 Discussion of 4.5 Demonstration and role play using physical assessment schedule	Own families Out-patient department Hospitals units Task: Do physical examination
5. Mental status examination 5.1 Components 5.2 Dealing with problems	Reading on 5.1 Demonstration of 5.2	Neurological unit Old age home Task: do mental status examination

The process of designing units starts by establishing what learning will take place as a result of this unit, with the intention of identifying desirable results (outcomes or competencies). Questions such as what should the students know and be able to do on completion of this module, what is desirable from the learners in terms of knowledge, skills and attitude on completion of this module, are important at this stage. Once the desirable results are established, assessments should be designed and be aligned with the learning goals. This stage entails determining acceptable evidence of learning (assessment criteria), establishing how one will know if the students have achieved the desired results and met the standards. What will be accepted as convincing evidence that the students have achieved the expected or desirable outcomes must be established. The last stage focuses on designing learning experiences and making decisions about appropriate teaching methods. The starting point at this stage is establishing the prerequisite knowledge and skills needed by the students in order to perform effectively and achieve desirable outcomes. A decision is made regarding what needs to be taught (content) and learned by the students. This includes the knowledge, skills, attitudes and values which are specific to the desired results in that particular unit. The planners should also establish how teaching and learning of the required competency should be done in order to achieve the desired results, what resources (human and material) are best suited to facilitate the achievement of desirable outcomes and whether the overall design is coherent and effective to achieve the set outcomes. Teaching in OBE is viewed as a means to an end; it is a tool used to facilitate the achievement of required competencies.

When designing mini modules (units) within a module, each unit should stipulate a specific outcome expected on completion of that unit, the learning resources required to develop the expected competence, a variety of teaching/learning methods to be used, ranging from learning through experience (hands-on), demonstrations, video tapes, interactive CD ROMs, lectures, etc., clinical placements and relevant and/or recommended learning materials, human resources to be consulted, specific dates and times of those learning experiences and a wide range of methods of assessments, including the dates of assessments and/or evaluation.

The variety of teaching and assessment methods used indicates that there is a lot of flexibility in OBE, especially because OBE is based on a premise that the same results may be achieved through different ways. Table 12.4 presents an example of a unit titled 'assessing the health status of individuals'. This unit is part of the nursing assessment module presented above. The competence expected in this module is that 'the nurse should be capable of assessing the health behaviour, physical and mental health status of an individual of any age'.

Table 12.4 Assessing the health status of an individual

Specific outcomes	Learning resources	Assessment criteria
1. Assess the health behaviour and the underlying knowledge and beliefs of an adult with regard to own basic needs	**Lecture** Basic human needs of an adult and their assessment Monday 08.00–09.30 **Demonstration** Interview – re: health behaviour with an adult Monday 10.00–11.30 (Room 207) **Video in library** Assessing nutritional habits **Expert practitioner** Sr S Hlabi, Geriatric Unit, Umbilo Hospital Sr P Thomas, Adult Medical Unit **Clinical Placement** Minimum 4 hours in a PHC clinic – Nutritional assessment Minimum 4 hours in adult medical unit – General assessment of an adult Minimum 4 hours in Geriatric Unit – Assessing mobility and intake and output	Accurately records health practices of adults, giving reasons in terms of beliefs and knowledge **Evaluation dates** – **Friday 7 February** – **Friday 10 March** – **Friday 17 March**

Assessment of learning in OBE

Assessment should be linked to learning and instruction and used to facilitate the development of the learner. The main purpose of assessment is twofold, to identify areas and degree of competence and to provide feedback for learning. It is also used to determine the basis for remedial action, whether to allow students to progress to the next level or whether to keep them at the same level. OBE assessment differs from measurement which is aimed at measuring the learner's status. It helps the students determine where they are in the process of learning and where they need to be in order to achieve their outcomes.

OBE assessment should cater for three areas of competence: foundational, applied and flexible competence, and thus it requires integrated methods of assessment. Integrated assessment refers to the use of a number of assessment methods to assess the learner's competence, and to assist in the process of making a decision about whether a learner is competent or not. Some of the alternative assessment methods which could be integrated include observations, demonstrations, self-directed projects, group work, portfolios, teacher-constructed performance tasks, projects and self-assessment. Assessment options for the cognitive domain include written assignments, observation of classroom discussions, written or oral problem-solving exercises, essays, portfolios and many other options. The affective domain can be assessed through observation of discussions, observation of interaction with clients and other members of the team, interviews, learning projects which require students to take a certain position, essays, learner debates, and many other options. The psychomotor domain is assessed through performance of authentic tasks directly related to real-life problems. Performance tasks may range from demonstrations to projects, development of oral or visual presentations, all dealing with real-life problems. Planning and designing assessments require the teacher to establish what the learners need to know and be able to do, how they will demonstrate what they have learned, what resources must be available to ensure that all learners succeed and how the teacher can structure or pace his/her teaching so that learners are prepared to perform well. Answers to these questions should serve as a guide to assessment of learning.

As outcomes-based assessment has a critical role to play in the whole learning process; there are vital questions to be asked when considering the most effective process of assessing the learning outcomes and these include:

- Does the assessment focus on what is important, what is of value, and what learners will need in order to succeed in future?
- Does the assessment process serve learners by giving them useful information that will make a meaningful difference to them?
- Are the results used fairly, meaningfully and in a manner that empowers the learners?
- Does the assessment process incorporate multiple strategies that encourage the learners to demonstrate learning outcomes through a variety of acceptable means?
- Does the assessment process provide the teacher with enough information about the effectiveness of his/her teaching? (Department of Education, 1997d).

In OBE, assessment should facilitate the growth of the learners. Therefore assessment intended for development of learners should:

1. help the learner to monitor his or her own development. Feedback can be given on a continuous basis. A learning dialogue should be established throughout the learning process
2. help the learners monitor the discrepancy between their self-perceptions or self-assessments and external information about their competence

3. be to the benefit of the learner instead of the institution. The learner should be the one who profits from this information and who should be able to utilize it for increased awareness

4. reflect the competence acquired, namely, the performance itself, in the sense that process as well as products are documented (in Tilema et al., 2000).

The assessment process in OBE is different from assessment in content-based education because there is a change in the role of the learner and the assessment is planned as early as possible in the curriculum, before planning the methods of instruction to facilitate the development of the learners. Learners become active partners in assessment. They learn to judge their own work and adopt goals for self-improvement, with the assistance of the teacher serving as an expert and providing feedback to the learners. The learners are involved in self-assessment as well as in peer and group assessment, to monitor their growth.

Just like all assessment, assessment in OBE should meet certain assessment principles. The assessment procedures should be (a) valid, (b) reliable, (c) fair, and (d) reflect the knowledge and skills that are most important for students. Moreover, the assessment should tell teachers and individual students something that they don't already know. They should allow for the students to be stretched to the limits of their understanding and ability, to apply their knowledge, both comprehensive and explicit. They should support every student's opportunity to learn things that are important and contribute to desirable results; and, because learners are individuals, assessments should allow this individuality to be demonstrated. This evidence of individuality is facilitated through the use of integrated methods or a variety of assessment methods.

In OBE assessment should be motivating to the learners, it should build their confidence and guide them in their learning. Positive feedback, constructive advice or criticism, encouragement and support, as well as helping the learners to improve their self-assessment skills could all be useful. Demotivating assessment, on the other hand, contributes little or nothing to the development of the learner. For example, educators should not make assessment comments which leave learners unclear of what they do not know or what they need to improve, and make the learners feel hopeless. Assessments where the ranking of the learners' marks classify the majority of learners as average or weak with very few, if any, graded as high achievers, lead to learners internalizing poor perceptions about themselves. Such systems covertly teach them that they are under-performers and that that is what is expected from them (Department of Education and Training 1997c). It is recommended that ranking or grading should be accompanied by detailed comments about the learner's performance as a way of substantiating the reason for poor performance. Assessment in OBE is used as an instrument to facilitate learning, therefore it should be well planned and be constructive to the learners, in order to serve its purpose.

Conclusion

Dynamics in the workplaces and in society have contributed to the paradigm shift to outcomes-based education. Although the introduction of OBE has resulted in a number of concerns, the benefits of this approach to education outweigh its disadvantages, especially because it prepares the graduates for service.

Developing an outcomes-based curriculum might pose as a challenge but it is a worthwhile exercise. Assessment is central to learning, as it is used to facilitate the learners' development and to evaluate the competence of the learner during and on completion of the programme.

Points for discussion

1. Does the strong focus on workplace demands pose a threat to the leadership and independent thinking of nurse educators?
2. How can you make sure that the nurses from this kind of programme are not only technically skilled, but lack in-depth knowledge and professional values?

References

Bonville, W. (1996) *What is Outcomes-based Education*. Online. Available at: hptt://www.new-jerusalem...education/WhatIsOBE.html. (Accessed November, 2003).

Department of Education (1997a) *Curriculum 2005 Implementing OBE – 4: Philosophy: Lifelong Learning for the 21st Century*. Cape Town, South Africa: CTP Book Printers.

Department of Education (1997b) *Curriculum 2005 Implementing OBE – 1: Classroom practice. Lifelong Learning for the 21st Century*. Cape Town, South Africa: CTP Book Printers.

Department of Education (1997c) *Curriculum 2005 Implementing OBE – 2: Assessment: Lifelong Learning for the 21st Century*. Cape Town, South Africa: CTP Book Printers.

Department of Education (1997d) *Outcomes-based Education: A Teacher's Manual*. Cape Town, South Africa. Kagiso Publishers.

Harden, R. M., Crosby, J.R. and Davis, M.H. (1999) AMEE Guide No 14: Outcomes-based education: Part 1 – An introduction to outcome-based education. *Medical Teacher*, 21(1): 7–14.

Malan, S. P. T. (2000) The new paradigm of outcomes-based education in perspective. *Journal of Family Ecology and Consumer Sciences*, 28: 22–28.

Prozesky, D. (2003) *Developing a Course Curriculum*. Online. Available at: hptt://www.jceh.co.uk/journal/36_6. asp

Spady, W. G. (1994a). Choosing outcomes of significance. *Educational Leadership*, 51(5): 18–22.

Spady, W. (1994b) *Outcomes-based Education: Critical Issues and Answers*. Arlington, VA: American Association of School Administrators.

Spady, W. G. and Marshall, K. J. (1991) Transformational outcomes-based educational curriculum restructuring. *Educational Researcher*, 6(2): 9–15.

Tillema, H. H., Kessells, J. W. M. and Meijers, F. (2000) Competencies as building blocks for the integrated assessment with instruction in vocational education: a case from Netherlands. *Assessment and Evaluation in Higher Education*, 25(3): 265–280.

Recommended reading

McDaniel, E. A., Felder, B. D., Gordon, L., Hrutka, M. E. and Quinn, S. (2000) New faculty roles in learning outcomes education: the experiences of four models and institutions. *Innovative Higher Education*, 25(2): 143–157.
The article describes how four American universities implemented outcomes-based programmes. It is written in the form of interviews with a person from each setting, and throws light on different approaches and ideas.

Chapter 13

A curriculum for interprofessional learning

Mouza Suwaileh and Nomthandazo S Gwele

Introduction

The world is continuously facing challenges, especially in health care. The increasing diversity of the population, and the complexity of health problems call for the revision of the delivery of health care and consequently of the education of health professionals. One of the innovative approaches in health professional education which has recently become popular in addressing these challenges, is interprofessional learning or IPL.

Interprofessional learning is often used interchangeably with terms such as interdisciplinary education, shared learning, multiprofessional learning (MPL) and transprofessional education. The philosophical underpinning of this approach addresses collaboration, team work and learning together (Harden, 1998). Interprofessional learning is defined as an educational approach which includes at least two professions or disciplines, collaborating in the learning process with the goal of fostering interprofessional interactions. The ultimate goal is enhancing the practice of the disciplines involved. This approach has to be based on mutual understanding and respect for the actual and potential contributions of the disciplines (American Association of Colleges of Nursing, 2002).

There is general agreement in the literature that the provision of effective health care demands collaboration and team work. These are the core values of IPL. Interprofessional education, therefore, involves the collaboration and inter-active learning between learners from different professions. Its explicit aim is to examine each other's roles for the purpose of improving collaborative practice.

Characteristics of IPL

IPL can be implemented in pre-registration and post-registration programmes. It usually encompasses only a part of the total programme, since all professions have to address their unique learning separately. Parsell and Bligh (1999) identified the following dimensions of IPL, which have to be considered when designing an IPL module.

- *The relationships among various professional groups:* This dimension deals with values, attitudes and beliefs. It includes the professional identities, prejudices, stereotypical views of each other's professions, the historical status and the knowledge base of each of the professions involved.
- *Collaboration and teamwork:* This dimension focuses on the skills and knowledge needed to implement and engage in the collaborative learning successfully. These skills are centred on course design, teaching and learning strategies, resources, assessment and evaluation.
- *Roles and responsibilities:* These refer to what people actually do or what roles they play in the provision of holistic care to address the problems of clients. They include the coordination of these roles through collaboration and teamwork.
- *The outcomes:* The benefits to patients, professional practice and personal growth as a result of the IPL experience make up this dimension.

Based on this framework, Parsell and Bligh (1999) developed an instrument to measure student readiness for IPL in all four dimensions, and called it the Readiness for Inter-professional Learning Scale (RIPLS). When Horsburgh et al. (2001) used this scale to describe the attitude of medical, nursing and pharmacy students to shared learning, they found that attitudes were generally positive. Students believed that competence in team work skills and collaboration is important for holistic care. The perceptions about when the IPL should be implemented, however, showed greater variations.

The rationale for IPL

Rooted in the theoretical foundations of holistic care, IPL is aimed at providing patient- or client-centred care from a variety of professionals, for maximizing patient and/or client outcomes. The basic premise is that most health problems are multidimensional in nature, encompassing economic, social, spiritual consequences and/or needs. Hence it is believed that it is not feasible for any one professional, irrespective of the quality of her/his education and training, to cater for all these dimensions (Cyphert and Cunningham, 2001). In the UK, IPL has a long history. The call for IPL has permeated the national health policy frameworks in the UK for over 30 years. It is envisaged that IPL has the potential to facilitate interprofessional collaboration in health care and thus reduce fragmentation, with resultant improvement in patient outcomes (Reeves and Mann, 2003).

In 1988 the World Health Organization (WHO) issued a report that referred to IPL as one of the key initiatives to achieve the goal of 'Health for All'. The report called for collaboration and team work amongst health professionals in primary, secondary and rehabilitative care settings. They made the point that working together would be enhanced by learning together. In response, a number of schools initiated IPL initiatives.

There is general agreement in the literature that the benefits of IPL include:

- increasing the understanding of each other's expectations, roles and responsibilities
- gaining knowledge and skills that are appropriate to the workplace
- the exploration of various strategies to enhance collaboration and team work
- improved communication within and between professional groups (Carpenter, 1995; Parr et al., 2000; Parsell and Bligh, 1999).

Research on evaluation of IPL has, however, focused mainly on changes in attitudes, knowledge and skills, rather than the impact on quality of patient care and health outcomes.

It is not easy to implement IPL programmes. The following challenges have been described in such projects, using the classification system of the American Association of Colleges of Nursing (AACN):

- *Philosophical and sociological:* This group includes gender and class differences between professions, problems with commitment to the innovative approach and differences in the professions' focus and mission. Parsell and Bligh (1999) saw the problem of changing the attitudes of professionals as the most crucial problem in this kind of programme.
- *Organizational and structural:* Differences in scheduling and timing of each programme, variations in the levels of students, inadequate and insufficient clinical sites and/or facilities such as small group rooms, geographical distribution and budgeting constraints are included here. There are also differences in the size of student groups, and inconsistencies in teaching and assessment methods.
- *Academic and professional:* Here the challenges include role reversal and overlap, risk to professional identity, lack of or a need for faculty preparation, identification and selection of core courses and shared experiences, selection of various disciplines to be involved in the shared learning and identification and training of qualified mentors/preceptors (AACN, 2002; Horsburgh *et al.*, 2001; Parsell and Bligh, 1999).

The problems seem to be particularly severe in pre-registration programmes, with the result that less activity has been seen in this area than in post-registration programmes (Pirrie *et al.*, 1998). Nevertheless, IPL does seem to be an endeavour worth the trouble.

Models of IPL

Although literature abounds on IPL, there seems to be paucity of literature dealing specifically with models of IPL. A few could be discerned from the literature, however. These include delivery mode models and those that focus on IPL as development. Whatever the model used, the key element is the coming together of different professions for the purpose of learning together.

A stage-model of IPL

The basic premise on which the stage model of IPL is based is that the development of interprofessional skills, such as collaborative team work, understanding and appreciation of the roles of the various members of the interprofessional team and managing conflict is a process and not an event. Harden (1998) described interprofessional education as a continuum with the following stages: going from isolation to awareness to consultation to nesting (small units work together) to temporal coordination to shared teaching to correlation to complementary teaching and then finally to interprofessional education and transprofessional education.

Delivery mode-focused models

Four types of delivery-focused models of IPL are identifiable in the literature. These are the seminar, conference, event and clinical models. These models are aimed at helping learners integrate theory and practice, develop interprofessional knowledge and skills, engage in interprofessional practice and develop a healthy sense of self.

The seminar and conference models are largely classroom based models which use a variety of teaching strategies such as simulations, role plays, case studies and/or problem-oriented learning (Jacobs, 2001). The strength of these models is that they provide students with a relatively safe environment in which to practise taking responsibility for patient management and treatment. Similarly, application of interprofessional skills, such as communication, collaboration, negotiation and conflict management within a simulation environment often do not change patient outcomes. Although inadvertent outcomes with colleagues are a possibility, the consequence of unplanned consequences of the learning experiences are not as threatening in a classroom setting as in a real clinical environment.

The seminar model has its shortcomings. Application of theory to practice is not necessarily achieved, since environments are just that, simulated environments. The model does not really afford the learners with an opportunity to experience whether or not interprofessional work is feasible in the real world of healthcare practice. Once the students are placed in clinical settings, either as students or as beginning professionals, they soon learn that what seemed easy and manageable in the classroom, might not be so clear cut in the clinical world (Jacobs, 2001).

Event-based IPL programmes are characterized by one-off workshops or a series of workshops or conferences which draw a number of participants from different professions to discuss on a similar theme or topics of interest to all participating professions. An example of an event-focused IPL model would be an annual continuing education meeting of critical care practitioners involving nurses, doctors and emergency care practitioners. The real benefit of this model is that it offers an opportunity for the students to share their knowledge and skills whilst learning with and from each other without putting great demands for change in practice setting on participants. The following is an example of an event-based IPL.

An example from Bahrain

The College of Medicine and Medical Science, Arabian Gulf University, provides medical training in Bahrain, and the College of Health Sciences provides nursing training. Both of these institutions are situated in Manama and are leading higher education institutions in the Gulf region. Although both faculties believe in the importance of teamwork and the value of IPL, the fact is that the training takes place in two different institutions. This organizational factor has limited contact between both staff and students in the past.

In 2003, however, the two schools initiated a series of IPL activities to bridge this gap. The first IPL project chosen was a problem-based learning workshop, during which groups of two medical and two nursing students each tackled problem scenarios around ethical issues. The objectives were to bring together medical students and nursing students in collaborative learning, to improve the understanding of the ethical issues facing the professions indicate how these are viewed by different professions, and to develop shared meanings and values. The day-long workshop was facilitated by one teacher from medicine and one from nursing. The results were positive, with students experiencing enhanced inter-professional communication and team work, and a greater appreciation for each other's roles.

This initiative was followed by another collaborative workshop along similar lines around the topic of complementary and alternative health care, held in October 2003. Both of these workshops fed into a third collaborative project – students and faculty from the two professions presented papers together at two PHC conferences. Clearly, the IPL project has gained momentum, and has benefited both faculty and students.

The clinical model is the most commonly used approach to interprofessional education in the health professions (Jacobs, 2001; Richardson et al., 1997). Clinical IPL involves placing a group of students from different professions in the same clinical learning setting, with a view to enhancing collaborative work among them. Expected learning objectives for the placement are developed jointly by the faculty from all participating professions.

The strength of this model is the immediate application of theory to practice in real clinical situations. The concrete experience of working together in the provision of health care provides the learners with deeper understanding of the theory underpinning both interprofessional and uniprofessional education depending, of course, on the timing of the clinical learning experience. Furthermore, inaccuracies and entrenched stereotypes about other professions and clients and application of learned interprofessional skills are not only confronted through guided discussion and reflection in the case of the former, or practised within the protected laboratory environment in the case of the latter. Instead, the clinical model forces the learners to become aware of their preconceived ideas and stereotypes as well as to resolve them in order for any effective collaborative work to occur (Jacobs, 2001). The development of interprofessional skills in such a model, therefore, seems to be more by intuition and trial and error on the part of the learners. Ideally, however, students should be guided by their facilitators during the early stages of placement to ensure that they gain confidence in themselves and their ability to assume their respective roles in the care of patients and/or clients.

A mixed-mode model

A mixed-mode model seems to be one of the frequently used approaches to IPL. A mixed-mode model combines classroom learning with clinical learning. Learners from different professions register for an interprofessional module. Such a module or course is planned so that students from all participating professions are able to participate meaningfully, both in the classroom and in the clinical learning setting. A number of authors caution that IPL should not be equated with students from different professions taking the same course. An IPL course should be designed with the aim of achieving the educational goals of IPL. It should create space for learners to interrogate theory and practice, get to know each profession's roles in health care and identify uniprofessional strengths and limitations so as to be able to make informed judgements and insightful choices in shared and collaborative practice.

Similarly, clinical learning should be guided by clearly defined learning outcomes that encourage collaborative work. Selected clinical learning environments should provide rich learning experiences to allow students from all participating professions an opportunity to engage fully with interprofessional practice. For instance, studies involving teams of nursing, social work, medical students and students from other health professions would be better placed in acute care or outpatient departments, rather than in clinics. There is very little that medical students do in primary healthcare settings in developing countries. Medical students might not find such a clinical learning experience interesting for them as members of an interprofessional team.

Development and implementation

There are few clear guidelines in the literature on how and when IPL should be implemented. The AACN (2002) indicated in a recent report that a limited number of nursing schools include some interprofessional activities either in the classroom or in the clinical setting.

Key factors in developing and implementing IPL

Reeves and Mann (2003) identify four key factors in the development of IPL. According to these authors conceptual, operational, educational and evaluative factors determine the success and effectiveness of IPL.

Conceptual factors

The multiplicity of conceptions of IPL demands that those planning to embark on this educational approach make a concerted effort to arrive at a common understanding of the phenomenon. Clarity on aims is just as important as clarity on terminology. In addition, issues surrounding the cost of IPL to the institution and the learners must be investigated and analysed.

Operational factors

Operational factors to be considered include decisions regarding recruitment of management group, inclusion of key staff and setting aside time for planning, including negotiations with professional regulatory bodies if necessary (Reeves and Mann, 2003). The role of the management team is that of facilitating the change process. Effective team-work is a function of facilitative leadership. Leadership in interprofessional education, however, cannot be bestowed based on tradition, nor is it to be seen as independent of the context and constant. Leadership in collaborative teamwork is determined by the demands of the particular situation and the requisite knowledge and skills pertaining to what needs to be done. Hence, facilitative rather than authoritative leadership is recommended in IPL (Horder, 2000).

Educational factors

The significance of skilled facilitators in IPL cannot be over-emphasized. A true IPL experience cannot be neutral with regard to interprofessional issues. Facilitators need to be skilled in facilitating passionate discussions between professions. Unless skilfully managed, these debates might lead to conflict and/or silencing or marginalizing other voices. A facilitator who is skilled in questioning and probing as well as managing the process is invaluable in IPL classrooms and clinical learning settings. Recruiting and training facilitators who are willing to commit time and self to the process are key elements in developing an IPL curriculum. Barr describes the requisites for effective facilitation in IPL as:

- in-depth understanding of interactive methods
- commitment to IPL
- knowledge of group dynamics
- confidence and flexibility to creatively use professional differences within groups (cited in Reeves and Mann, 2003: 312).

The educational objectives of IPL demand interactive teaching/learning approaches, such as group discussions, case-based learning, problem-based learning, debates and inquiry-based learning (Reeves and Mann, 2003; Richardson et al., 1997). It is important that the teaching/learning environment should create a platform for students to debate and discuss issues related to interprofessional learning. Such an environment should make it clear to the student that every voice counts and that it is not important that everyone agrees with everyone on all that is discussed but that it is essential that differences of opinion be acknowledged and respected.

Evaluative factors

A systematic review carried out by Zwarenstein et al. (2002) on the effects of IPL on interprofessional practice and healthcare outcomes yielded a total of 1042 studies, none of which met the requirements for rigorous scientific analysis on which evidence for best practice could be drawn. There is a need for planned systematic and scientific evaluation of IPL programmes in order for those adopting the model to justify the time, cost and the over-extension of clinical learning facilities resulting from a large number of students needing access to similar resources at the same time. Reeves and Mann (2003) recommend multi-method, longitudinal research studies for monitoring and evaluating IPL.

Steps in the process of developing an IPL curriculum

The steps in the process of curriculum development need a considerable degree of modification when IPL is being included.

The context of the curriculum

The faculty of all the professions involved needs to create an environment conducive to the successful implementation of change. They have to support an educational philosophy which encourages questioning, initiative, problem-solving and reflective approaches to teaching and learning, since these elements are inherent in the IPL experience. To promote such an educational environment, teachers should be given opportunities for professional and personal growth. Visits to successful programmes, the exchange of success stories from their own teaching life and the sharing of problems they have experienced or are experiencing create a climate of supportive collegiality (Dockling, 1987).

During the phase of curriculum development when the context is established and foundations are laid, the health professionals have to reach consensus about whether IPL is necessary and why they are doing it. It is often valuable to involve stakeholders such as students and clients in these discussions, since they might bring a stronger consumer orientation to the discussions. The group should clarify for themselves what they aim to achieve with the IPL for each group of students.

Planning the macro- or micro-curriculum

In terms of the macro-curriculum, the academics from all participating professions have to decide where the IPL would fit into their own programmes. It is ideal that students are more or less on the same level of their programmes when they learn together. If the IPL experience takes place early in the professional programme, it might have a positive influence on the learning in the rest of the programme. Immersing students in IPL early in their professional education is, however, not without its own problems. Interprofessional education is about different professions contributing equally, as demanded by the health status of the patient or situation involved. Students without the requisite knowledge and skills to provide competent uniprofessional care have very little to offer in an interprofessional experience. Professional identities and competencies need to be fully developed for meaningful collaborative work. A number of authors warn that early immersion may in fact result in the opposite of what IPL seeks to achieve. It might entrench feelings of inferiority, superiority and stereotypes about other professions. For this reason, it is recommended that students in the senior years of their professional programmes are best suited for IPL. It is hoped that at a later stage of their educational careers, students would be competent in their own professional roles and responsibilities so as to be able to participate and contribute meaningfully in collaborative patient care (Jacobs, 2001). Furthermore, it might be easier for students to learn together when they are more sure of their own roles and comfortable in these roles.

Once the decision has been made about when the IPL will take place, and how long it will last, the setting has to be chosen. Students can share learning in the classroom, in a hospital, in a PHC setting or in a community. The content of the module(s) will be determined by both the level of the students, and the setting in which it takes place. The most successful topics or content are those that allow for distinct professional roles and which demand team-work (Harden, 1998).

The teaching/learning approach also has to be chosen. Students can be given a community-based task, such as running a volunteer PHC clinic. The task may also be of an academic nature, for instance planning and doing a research project together, or organizing a faculty research day. The group must also identify how the teachers of all the professions will be involved. Shared learning ideally goes hand-in-hand with shared teaching. An IPL experience run by the faculty of one profession only loses much of its impact.

Finally, decisions have to be made about the evaluation of the IPL experience. Students may be evaluated as individuals or as groups. The evaluation should be related to the outcomes of the IPL learning experience, and should ideally involve teachers from all the professions involved.

Providing for resources

The planning group should identify what additional resources would be necessary for the IPL, and make sure these resources are made available. Resources might include small group classrooms for groups to meet, funding for transport to clinical sites or to another educational institution, computer systems that 'talk' to each other, or shared library resources. The early involvement of key decision-makers should prove valuable at this stage.

Implementation

Crucial to successful implementation is coordination between the different professional groups. It might be a good idea to pilot test the curricular outcomes, teaching approach and evaluation instruments on a small scale before general implementation (Harriet et al., 2003). It is important that the teaching team serve as role models for team work and cooperation for the students, and this demands frequent and open communication, regular scheduled and minuted meetings and adequate attention to detail.

Conclusion

Although much emphasis is currently being placed on IPL, it is essential that the outcomes of this approach be more thoroughly evaluated. Nevertheless the AACN recommended in 2002 that schools of nursing increase the cooperative learning of nursing students from different levels (undergraduate and postgraduate) as well as different fields of nursing, and also increase interprofessional learning. Such suggestions need to be tested in order to guide curriculum decisions about cooperative learning.

Points for discussion

1. What do you see as the most problematic aspect of IPL in your own setting?
2. Why would IPL be a risk to professional identity, as the AACN says?

References

American Association of Colleges of Nursing (2002) *Inter-disciplinary Education and Practice: Position Statements*. Online. Available at: http://www.aacn.nche.edu/ Publications/positions/interdisk.htm (accessed May 2004).

Carpenter, J. (1995) Interprofessional education for medical and nursing students: evaluation of a programme. *Medical Education*, 29: 265–272.

Cyphert, F. R. and Cunningham, L. L. (2001) Interprofessional education and practice: A future agenda. *Theory into Practice, 24*(2): 153–156.

Docking, S. (1987) Curriculum innovation. In: P. Allan and M. Jolley (eds) *The Curriculum in Nursing Education*. London: Croom Helm.

Harden, R. M. (1998). AMEE Guide No. 12: Multiprofessional education: Part 1: Effective multiprofessional education: A three-dimensional perspective. *Medical Teacher, 20*(5): 402–408.

Harriet, B., Cummings, D. M. and Dreyfus, K. S. (2003) Evolution of an interdisciplinary curriculum. *Journal of Allied Health, 32*(4): 285–292.

Horder, J. (2000) Leadership in a multiprofessional context. *Medical Education*, 34: 203–205.

Horsburgh, M., Lamdin R. and Williamson, E. (2001) Multiprofessional learning: The attitudes of medical, nursing and pharmacy students to shared learning. *Medical Education*, 35: 876–883.

Jacobs, L. A. (2001) Interprofessional clinical education and practice. *Theory into Practice*, 24(2): 116–123.

Parr, R. M., Bryson, S. and Ryan, M. (2000) Shared learning – a collaborative education and training initiative for community pharmacists and general medical practitioners. *Pharmaceutical Journal*, 264(7077): 35–38.

Parsell, G. and Bligh, J. (1999) The development of a questionnaire to assess the readiness of health care students for inter-professional learning (RIPLS). *Medical Education*, 33: 95–100.

Pirrie, A., Wilson, V., Harden, R.M. and Elsegood, J. (1998) Promoting cohesive practice in health care. *Medical Teacher*, 20: 409–416.

Reeves, S. and Mann, S. L. (2003) Key factors to developing and delivering interprofessional education. *International Journal of Therapy and Rehabilitation*, 10(7): 310–313.

Richardson, J., Montemuro, M., Cripps, D., Mohide, E. A. and Macpherson, A. S. (1997) Educating students for interprofessional teamwork in the clinical placement setting. *Educational Gerontology, 23*: 669–693.

Zwarenstein, M., Reeves, S., Barr, S., Hammick, M., Koppel, I. and Atkins, J. (2002) *Interprofessional education: effects on professional practice and health care outcomes, Cochrane Review*. Oxford: The Cochrane Library Update Software.

Recommended reading

Harden, R. M. (1998) AMEE Guide No. 12: Multiprofessional education: Part 1: Effective multiprofessional education: A three-dimensional perspective. *Medical Teacher,* **20**(5): 402–408.

A useful article for implementers of IPL.

Horsburg, M., Lamdin, R. and Williamson, E. (2003) Multiprofessional learning: the attitudes of medical, nursing, and pharmacy students to shared learning. *Medical Teacher,* **35**: 876–883.

This article is descriptive in nature, and illustrates one way of evaluating this kind of curriculum.

Chapter 14

Conclusion

There is always more to be said on a topic such as curriculum development, which has many facets, many configurations and many processes. No single text will ever be complete, but we believe this one is adequate to support nurse educators who want to embark on major curriculum revision. To speed you on your way, we would like to conclude with a few pieces of advice we canvassed from the contributors. This is the one thing each one of them would like the curriculum team to keep in mind.

Leana: We have a saying in Afrikaans 'Haas jou langsaam' which translates into 'Hurry up slowly'. When embarking on major curriculum change, you have to move fast, since such a change takes so long to have an effect. Your first graduate from a new 4-year programme will only be produced 4 years from implementation date! Nevertheless, you also have to go slowly. You have to give yourself enough time to explore possibilities, think them through, prepare your whole school for the change, make sure your plans are coherent and that your staff can actually do what is asked of them, and put all the paperwork in place. All this takes time. So, go forward fast, but do it slowly!

I know this was supposed to be one piece of advice, but here is another one; when considering an external person to facilitate the curriculum change process, I would like to mention a few considerations. It is useful to have a person who uses the same language as your school teaches in. This allows the expert to become familiar with your system by reading your documents, and it allows for better understanding than through translators. A second consideration is to use a person who comes from a similar setting. It may be difficult for a person from a resource-rich system to assist a resource-poor system to overcome its barriers, since the person has never faced such challenges. Similarly, it might be difficult for a person from a hospital-based programme to assist a school to develop a community-based programme. Therefore you should choose a person who knows the kind of programme you want to develop. Lastly, choose a person who is willing to be involved over a period of time, and not one who will come once only for a brief period, and then leave you to struggle on your own.

Thandi: The need for a visionary and facilitative leader is invaluable in ensuring effective and successful implementation. Teachers need to know that there is someone they can count on to guide the process, to anticipate problems and help them find solutions; someone who will champion their cause to those responsible for funding and allocation of resources. Asking teachers to do too much with too little does not augur well for curriculum development and implementation.

Curriculum change can be daunting for a number of teachers. The experience is fraught with feelings of uncertainty and anxiety for some. Monitoring and dealing with staff concerns during the curriculum development and the implementation process is one of the most important things a change agent will have to do. Curriculum change takes place in the classroom. Teachers are professionals in their own right, they have their own beliefs and values about the purpose of education and what is worthwhile nursing education. Involve them very early in the change process. Make them feel they own the change. This requires a concerted effort in staff capacity development. Literature abounds with accounts of failed innovations due to lack of capacity to implement new curriculum. Learning new ways of doing things takes time. Curriculum change agents must realize this and make a concerted effort to walk alongside the teachers as they begin their journey of discovery in an effort to learn the requisite knowledge and skills demanded by the introduction of a new curriculum.

Last but not the least; students are just as wary of change as the staff. Curriculum change that involves students assuming responsibility for their own learning, using alternative clinical placements, or any aspect of the curriculum that breaks away from tradition can be met with resistance from the students. Students want to know what effect the change will have on national and international recognition of their qualifications; they also want to know what the teachers will be doing, if they have to be self-directing in their learning. Unless students are part of the decision to change, sharing the vision and the philosophy underpinning a new and innovative curriculum, it would be very difficult for them to appreciate and accept a curriculum that requires more from them than is traditionally the case.

Fikile: Innovations in nursing education are imperative because of the dynamics in society and in the workplace. However, successful implementation of these innovations requires careful consideration of a number of issues. Among these issues is that change is accompanied by uncertainty, anxieties, fear and resistance, which could be avoided by the early involvement of staff in decision-making regarding the innovation and through proper planning and preparation for the proposed change. Secondly, as nursing education institutions are supposed to be working in collaboration with the health service and surrounding communities, the proposed change should be communicated with these stakeholders to make them part of the change process, especially because they will be involved in the teaching of students and they will be the consumers of the produced product. Thirdly, available resources should be adapted creatively to meet the needs for the change, as innovations might be heavy on resources. Lastly, the innovation should comply with the country's nursing education regulations and accreditation standards because the school is not preparing graduates for the sake of preparing them but for them to be able to render service competently to the community at large.

Henry: The process of curriculum development and review is dynamic. As a tool to guarantee the quality of an educational programme, the curriculum should always meet the criteria of a good standard, which include reliability, validity, clarity and being realistic. Therefore, it needs constant review whenever there are indications that due to one reason or the other, those criteria are not being met. A curriculum review should be done after carrying out an evaluation of the curriculum currently in use and the evaluation should include all the stakeholders, especially the graduates of the programme, but also the tutors/lecturers, the community being served, and management/policymakers. A team of subject experts and curriculum experts should constitute the review committee.

Marilyn: When introducing change, be sure to take academic staff along with you, i.e., academic staff must believe that: (a) change is necessary and (b) this is the most appropriate change. Find a champion, someone who has experience with the new element(s) and is willing to lead in the change process. For example, if you wish to semesterize a programme, find someone familiar with semesterized academic programmes. Pilot the change, for example, start with a small group such as 1 year of a programme or one department in a school, etc. Develop staff members as necessary to assist in implementation of the change. For example, if you are introducing change in delivery of a programme to a case- or problem-based approach academic staff members must be trained to use this process. Members of staff who have experience with a particular curriculum element (champions) should act as mentors for those without experience. Be sure that there is congruence among the elements of the curriculum, if there is incongruence it will be difficult implementing and embedding the change. Build in monitoring and evaluation processes into the plan for implementation of change.

In reviewing the advice, it is interesting to note what is repeated amongst the authors. Relevance seems to be an important aspect, as is the importance of 'taking people with you' on the journey of change. Similarly, making sure there is a person to lead the process is repeatedly mentioned. However much information is given in this text, many questions will arise during the process of curriculum change, which are not answered by the contributors to this book. We are sure that you will deal with these questions creatively and make a success of your project.

Index

Note: Page references in *italics* refer to tables or boxed material in the text